Helen Meehan

Symptom Management in Advanced Cancer

Lead Nurse Palliative Care

Second edition

Robert Twycross DM, FRCP, FRCR

Macmillan Clinical Reader in Palliative Medicine,
Oxford University
Consultant Physician, Sir Michael Sobell House,
Churchill Hospital, Oxford
Senior Research Fellow, St Peter's College, Oxford
Director, WHO Collaborating Centre for
Palliative Cancer Care, Oxford
Chairman, International School for Cancer Care

RADCLIFFE MEDICAL PRESS

Radcliffe Medical Press Ltd
18 Marcham Road, Abingdon, Oxon, OX14 1AA, UK

British Library Cataloguing in Publication Data

A catalogue record for this book is available from the British Library.

ISBN 1 85775 282 1

Library of Congress Cataloging-in-Publication Data is available.

Typeset by Advance Typesetting Ltd, Oxon
Printed and bound by Biddles Ltd, Guildford and King's Lynn

Contents

Preface

Symptom Management in Advanced Cancer represents the current practice of a doctor with over 26 years experience in palliative care. For greater detail, the reader is referred to more scholarly books, notably:

Twycross R (1994) *Pain Relief in Advanced Cancer*. Churchill Livingstone, Edinburgh

Doyle D, Hanks GW and MacDonald N (1997) *Oxford Textbook of Palliative Medicine*. (2nd edn) Oxford Medical Publications, Oxford

Symptom Management in Advanced Cancer is written primarily for doctors. It provides a framework of knowledge which will enable the clinician to develop a scientific approach to the management of symptoms in advanced cancer. The book will also be of interest and value to nurses working with cancer patients, particularly in palliative care.

International nonproprietary names (INNs) are used to increase the usefulness of the book; few proprietary names are included. Readers are directed to publications such as their own *National Formulary* and, in the USA, the *Physicians Desk Reference* to ascertain or confirm local options.

The contents of any textbook can never be wholly original. Over the years, much information and help has been received from colleagues, other professional contacts and pupils. Insights have also been obtained from many articles and books. I am particularly grateful to my colleagues at Sobell House for their help in reading draft chapters and giving much valuable advice; and to the Dietitians of the Oxford Radcliffe Hospital Trust; Mary Walding, Ward Sister with a special interest in bedsores; Catherine Meadows and Angie Perrin, Clinical Nurse Specialists in Stomatherapy; Karen Jenns, Clinical Nurse Specialist in Lymphoedema; Angela Williams, Research Nurse in Lymphoedema. I am also grateful to David Cole for his advice on skin care for patients undergoing radiotherapy, to Mark Churcher for advice about sympathetically maintained pain in cancer patients and to David Marshall-Searson for help in creating Figures 2.8, 8.2 and 10.1.

Table 8.6 is reproduced by kind permission of Claud Regnard and Oxford University Press. Figures 11.1, 11.2 and Plates 2,4 are reproduced by permission of ConvaTec; Plate 1 by permission of Jenny Millward; and Plate 3 by permission of George Cherry. Finally, I should like to thank Karen Allen for preparing the typescript for publication and Susan Brown, copy-editor, for her painstaking attention to detail.

Robert Twycross
September 1997

Drug names

For some drugs marketed in the UK, the International Nonproprietary Name (INN) differs from the British Approved Name (BAN). From January 1998, the use of BANs will be discontinued and all drugs marketed in the UK will be known by their INN.

More than 40 drugs have a BAN which is different from their corresponding INN; those relevant to palliative care are listed below.

BAN	INN
Adrenaline	Epinephrine
Amylobarbitone	Amobarbital
Bendrofluazide	Bendroflumethiazide
Benzhexol	Trihexyphenidyl
Benztropine	Benzatropine
Chlorpheniramine	Chlorphenamine
Dicyclomine	Dicycloverine
Dimethicone	Dimeticone
Frusemide	Furosemide
Hexamine hippurate	Methenamine hippurate
Indomethacin	Indometacin
Lignocaine	Lidocaine
Methotrimeprazine	Levomepromazine
Noradrenaline	Norepinephrine
Oestradiol	Estradiol
Oxethazaine	Oxetacaine
Phenobarbitone	Phenobarbital
Stilboestrol	Diethylstilbestrol
Trimeprazine	Alimemazine

Differences also exist between INNs and adopted names in the USA (USANs).

INN	USAN
Dimeticone[a]	Simethicone
Dextropropoxyphene	Propoxyphene
Glycopyrronium	Glycopyrrolate
Paracetamol	Acetaminophen
Pethidine	Meperidine

a   in some countries, dimeticone is called (di)methylpolysiloxane.

Note also that

• diamorphine (available only in the UK and Canada) = di-acetylmorphine = heroin

• hyoscine = scopolamine

• liquid paraffin = mineral oil.

All the drugs referred to in *Symptom Management in Advanced Cancer* are not universally available. Please check with your own National Formulary or drug compendium if in doubt.

List of abbreviations

General

BNF	British National Formulary
BP	British Pharmacopoeia
IASP	International Association for the Study of Pain
UK	United Kingdom
USA	United States of America
USP	United States Pharmacopoeia
WHO	World Health Organization

Medical

CNS	central nervous system
COPD	chronic obstructive pulmonary disease
COX	cyclo-oxygenase
CSF	cerebrospinal fluid
CT	computed tomography
5HT	5-hydroxytryptamine (serotonin)
H_1, H_2	histamine type 1, type 2 receptors
MAOI(s)	mono-amine oxidase inhibitor(s)
MRI	magnetic resonance imaging
NMDA	N-methyl D-aspartate
NSAID(s)	nonsteroidal anti-inflammatory drug(s)
PCA	patient controlled analgesia
PG(s)	prostaglandin(s)

RIMA(s)   reversible inhibitor(s) of mono-amine oxidase type A

SSRI(s)   selective serotonin re-uptake inhibitor(s)

Drug administration

b.d.   twice daily; alternative, b.i.d.

ED   epidural

IM   intramuscular

IT   intrathecal

IV   intravenous

m/r   modified release; alternative, slow release

nocte   at bedtime

o.d.   daily, once a day

p.c.   post cebus, after meals

PO   per os, by mouth

PR   per rectum, by rectum

q.d.s.   four times a day (per 24 h); alternative, q.i.d.

q4h, q6h   every 4 hours, every 6 hours etc.

SC   subcutaneous

SL   sublingual

stat   immediately

t.d.s.   three times a day (per 24 h); alternative, t.i.d.

Units

cm   centimetre(s)

cps   cycles per sec

Gy   Gray(s), a measure of radiation

g   gram(s)

h	hour(s)
Hg	mercury
IU	international unit(s)
kg	kilogram(s)
l	litre(s)
mcg	microgram(s)
mEq	milli-equivalent(s)
mg	milligram(s)
ml	millilitre(s)
mm	millimetre(s)
mmol	millimole(s)
min	minute(s)

1 General principles

Biopsychosocial care · Ethical considerations
Symptom management · As death approaches

Biopsychosocial care

Care of the dying extends far beyond pain and symptom management – important though these are. It includes supporting

- the patient as he adjusts to his decreasing physical ability and as he mourns in anticipation the loss of family, friends and all that is familiar
- the family as they adjust to the fact that one of them is dying.

Although psychologically demanding for doctors, nurses and other carers, it is potentially one of the most rewarding of their responsibilities. One of the keys to success is an attitude of partnership between the caring team and the patient and family (Table 1.1).

Table 1.1 Partnership with the patient

Courtesy in behaviour	Explaining
Politeness in speech	Agreeing priorities and goals
Not patronizing	Discussing treatment options
Being honest	Accepting treatment refusal
Listening	

To be maximally supportive, it is also necessary to show that you care about the patient as a person, and that you are not just concerned about physical symptoms. Beginning consultations with an open question is one way of doing this. For example:

'Where would you like to begin?'

'How are you feeling today?'

'How have you been coping since we last met?'

An enquiry from time to time about how the family is coping is also interpreted by the patient as an indication of your general interest and concern. Finally, at the end of the consultation, ask the patient if there are any questions he would like to ask you.

Ethical considerations

The ethics of palliative care are those of medicine in general. Doctors have a dual responsibility, namely to preserve life and to relieve suffering. At the end of life, relief of suffering is of even greater importance as preserving life becomes increasingly impossible.

Four cardinal principles[1]

- patient autonomy (respect for the patient as a person)
- beneficence (do good)
- nonmaleficence (minimize harm)
- justice (fair use of available resources).

The four cardinal principles need to be applied against a background of

- respect for life
- acceptance of the ultimate inevitability of death.

In practice, these comprise three dichotomies which need to be applied in a balanced manner. Thus

- the potential benefits of treatment must be balanced against the potential burdens
- striving to preserve life but, when biologically futile, providing comfort in dying
- individual needs are balanced against those of society.

Appropriate treatment

All patients must die eventually. Part of the art of medicine is to decide when sustaining life is essentially futile and, therefore, when to allow death to occur without further impediment. Thus, in palliative care, the primary aim of treatment is not to prolong life but to make the life which remains as comfortable and as meaningful as possible.

A doctor is not obliged legally or ethically to preserve life 'at all costs'. Rather, life should be sustained when from a biological point of view it is sustainable. Priorities change when a patient is clearly dying. There is no obligation to employ treatments if their use can best be described as prolonging the process of dying. A doctor has neither a duty nor the right to prescribe a lingering death.

It is not a question of to treat or not to treat but what is the most appropriate treatment given the patient's biological prospects and his personal and social circumstances? Appropriate treatment for an acutely ill patient may be inappropriate in the dying (Figures 1.1 and 1.2).

Nasogastric tubes, IV infusions, antibiotics, cardiac resuscitation and artificial respiration are all primarily support measures for use in acute or acute-on-chronic illnesses to assist a patient through the initial crisis towards recovery of health. To use such measures in patients who are close to death and in whom there is no expectation of a return to health is generally inappropriate (and therefore bad medicine).

Medical care is a continuum, ranging from complete cure at one end to symptom relief at the other. Many types of treatment span the entire spectrum, notably radiotherapy and, to a lesser extent, chemotherapy and surgery. It is

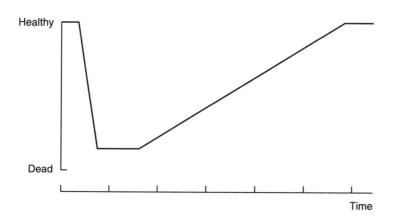

Figure 1.1 A graphical representation of acute illness. Biological prospects are generally good. Acute resuscitative measures are important and enable the patient to survive the initial crisis. Recovery is aided by the natural forces of healing; rehabilitation is completed by the patient on his own, without continued medical support.

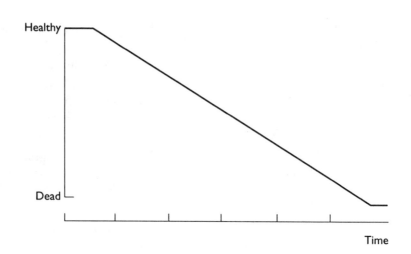

Figure 1.2 A graphical representation of terminal illness. Biological prospects progressively worsen. Acute and terminal illnesses are therefore distinct pathophysiological entities. Therapeutic interventions which can best be described as prolonging the distress of dying are futile and inappropriate.

important to keep the therapeutic aim clearly in mind with any form of treatment. In deciding what is appropriate, the key points are

- the patient's biological prospects
- the therapeutic aim and benefits of each treatment
- the adverse effects of treatment
- the need not to prescribe a lingering death.

Although the possibility of unexpected improvement or recovery should not be ignored, there are many occasions when it is appropriate to 'give death a chance'.

As a person becomes terminally ill, or severely limited physically and mentally as a result of senile decay, his interest in hydration and nutrition often becomes minimal. Because the natural outcome of both incurable progressive disease and advanced senility is death, these are circumstances in which it is wrong to force a patient to accept food and fluid. The patient's disinterest or positive disinclination should be seen as part of the process of letting go.

Symptom management

Attendance by the patient at several different outpatient clinics should be discouraged. Ideally, one team should co-ordinate, direct and explain all aspects of care. Further, both the patient and the family must know to whom they should turn in an emergency.

The scientific approach to pain and symptom management can be summarized as

- evaluation
- explanation
- individualized treatment
- supervision
- attention to detail.

Patients are often reluctant to bother their doctor about minor symptoms such as dry mouth, altered taste, anorexia, pruritus, cough and insomnia. Enquiries should be made from time to time rather than relying on spontaneous reports.

Evaluation

Evaluation must precede treatment

The cancer itself is not always the cause of a symptom. Further, some symptoms are caused by several factors. Causal factors include

- cancer
- treatment
- debility
- concurrent disorder.

Treatment depends on the underlying pathological mechanism

Even when the cancer is responsible, a symptom may be caused in different ways, e.g. vomiting from hypercalcaemia and vomiting from raised intracranial pressure. Treatment will vary accordingly.

Explanation

Explain the underlying mechanism(s) in simple terms

Treatment begins with an explanation by the doctor of the reason(s) for the symptom. This knowledge does much to reduce the psychological impact of the symptom on the sufferer, e.g. 'The shortness of breath is caused partly by the cancer itself and partly by the fluid at the base of the right lung. In addition, you are anaemic.'

If explanation is omitted, the patient may continue to think that his condition is shrouded in mystery. This is frightening because 'even the doctors don't know what's going on'.

Discuss treatment options with the patient

Whenever possible, the doctor and the patient should decide together on the immediate course of action. Few things are more damaging to a person's self-esteem than to be excluded from discussions about one's self.

Explain the treatment to the family

Discussion with close relatives generally enlists their co-operation and helps to re-inforce symptom management strategies. This is particularly important when the patient is at home. If actively involved in supporting the patient, the family have a right to be informed subject to the patient's approval. It is important, however, not to let the family take over. Whenever possible, the patient's wishes should prevail.

Individualized treatment

Decide priorities

Most patients with advanced cancer have multiple symptoms, e.g. pain, constipation, anorexia, weight loss, insomnia, anxiety – and possibly nausea, vomiting, lack of energy and dyspnoea as well. In the face of such a list, it may be difficult to know what to deal with first – unless the consultation began with an open question (see p.1). Even so, at some point it may be necessary to say to the patient:

> 'Today, we'll begin to deal with the pain, constipation, vomiting and insomnia. Then, next week, we can begin to think about some of your other symptoms – loss of appetite, lack of energy and so on.'

In the above example, pain is the prime focus. Treating (or preventing) constipation and vomiting is always integral to pain management. It means that most patients will need to take at least four different medications in addition to any long term medication for chronic conditions such as COPD or ischaemic heart disease.

Do not limit treatment to the use of drugs

- treatment may have a physical or a psychological focus, or both
- treatment may be drug or nondrug or both.

For example, pruritus is relieved in the majority of patients without resort to antihistamines. Aqueous cream applied to dry, itching skin several times a day and soap eliminated in favour of emulsifying ointment is frequently sufficient.

Prescribe drugs prophylactically for persistent symptoms

When treating a persistent symptom with a drug, it should be administered regularly on a prophylactic basis. The use of drugs as needed instead of regularly is the cause of much unrelieved distress.

Keep the treatment as straightforward as possible

When an additional drug is considered, ask the following questions:

'What is the treatment goal?'

'How can it be monitored?'

'What is the risk of adverse effects?'

'What is the risk of drug interactions?'

'Is it possible to stop any of the current medications?'

Written advice is essential

Precise guidelines are necessary to achieve maximum patient co-operation. 'Take as much as you like, as often as you like' is a recipe for anxiety, poor symptom relief and maximum adverse effects. The drug regimen should be written out in full for the patient and his family to work from (Figures 1.3 and 1.4). Times to be taken, names of drugs, reason for use (for pain, for bowels etc.) and dose (x ml, y tablets) should all be stated. Also the patient should be advised how to obtain further supplies, e.g. from his general practitioner.

SIR MICHAEL SOBELL HOUSE

Name   *Mary Smith*   **Date** *August 15, 1997*

TABLETS/ MEDICINES	2 am	On waking	10 am	2 pm	6 pm	Bedtime	PURPOSE
ORAMORPH (2 mg in 1 ml)		10 ml	10 ml	10 ml	10 ml	20 ml	pain relief
METOCLOPRAMIDE (10 mg tablet)		1	1	1	1	1	anti-sickness
FLURBIPROFEN (100 mg tablet)			1			1	pain relief
AMITRIPTYLINE (50 mg tablet)						1	for sleep and to help mood
CO-DANTHRUSATE (capsules)			2			2	for bowels

If troublesome pain   take extra 10 ml of ORAMORPH betweem regular doses

If bowels constipated   increase CO-DANTHRUSATE to 3 capsules twice a day

Figure 1.3   Take-home medication chart (q4h).

Seek a colleague's advice in seemingly intractable situations

No one can be an expert in all aspects of patient care. For example, the management of an unusual genito-urinary problem is likely to be enhanced by advice from a urologist or gynaecologist.

SIR MICHAEL SOBELL HOUSE

Name *John Bull*   **Date** *August 15, 1997*

TABLETS/MEDICINES	Breakfast	Midday meal	Evening meal	Bedtime	PURPOSE
ASILONE (suspension)	10 ml	10 ml	10 ml	10 ml	for hiccups
MORPHINE slow-release (100 mg tablet)	1			1	pain relief
FLURBIPROFEN slow-release (200 mg capsule)	1				pain relief
HALOPERIDOL (1.5 mg tablet)				1	anti-sickness
CO-DANTHRUSATE (capsules)	2			2	for bowels
TEMAZEPAM (20 mg tablet)				1	for sleeping

If troublesome pain   take liquid morphine (ORAMORPH 2 mg in 1 ml) 15 ml up to every 3 hours

If troublesome hiccup   take extra 10 ml of ASILONE up to every 2 hours

Figure 1.4   Take-home medication chart (q.d.s.).

Never say 'I have tried everything' or 'There is nothing more I can do'

It is generally possible to develop a repertoire of alternative measures. Although it is wise not to promise too much, it is important to re-assure the patient that you are going to stand by him and do all you can to help, e.g. 'No promises but we'll do our best.'

Instead of attempting immediately to relieve a symptom completely, be prepared to chip away at the problem a little at a time. When tackled in this way it is often surprising how much can be achieved with determination and persistence.

Supervision

Review! Review! Review!

It is often difficult to predict the optimum dose of a symptom relief drug, particularly opioids, laxatives and psychotropic drugs. Further, adverse effects put drug compliance in jeopardy. Arrangements must be made for continuing supervision and adjustment of medication.

It is sometimes necessary to compromise on complete relief in order to avoid unacceptable adverse effects. For example, anticholinergic effects such as dry mouth or visual disturbance may limit dose escalation. With inoperable bowel obstruction it may be better to aim to reduce the incidence of vomiting to once or twice a day rather than to seek complete relief.

Cancer is a progressive disease and new symptoms occur. These must be dealt with urgently.

Attention to detail

'Do not make assumptions.'

'To *ass-u-me* is to make an *ass* of *u* and *me*.'[2]

Attention to detail requires an inquisitive mind, one which repeatedly asks why:

'Why is this patient with breast cancer vomiting? She is not taking morphine; she is not hypercalcaemic. Why is she vomiting?'

'This patient with cancer of the pancreas has pain in the neck. It does not fit with the typical pattern of metastatic spread. Why does he have pain there?'

Attention to detail is important at every stage – in evaluation, explanation (e.g. avoid jargon, use simple language) and when planning and prescribing treatment (e.g. preparing written advice and drug regimens which are easy to follow).

Attention to detail is also necessary in the psychological, social and spiritual dimensions

- validate the patient's feelings, e.g. 'It's natural you should feel like that'
- respond to verbal cues, e.g. 'It's like Granny's illness' – 'What do you mean "It's like Granny's illness"?'
- reflect back the patient's question for clarification, e.g. 'I'm frightened, doctor' … 'What exactly is frightening you?'

Attention to detail makes all the difference to palliative care – without it success may be forfeited and patients suffer needlessly.

As death approaches

With increasing weakness, the patient is faced with the fact that death is inevitable and imminent. Support and companionship are of paramount importance at this time.

Weakness is commonly associated with drowsiness or the need to rest for more prolonged periods. Explanation is essential:

'This often happens in an illness like yours.'   [The doctor understands]

'When the body is short of energy it takes a lot more effort to do even simple jobs. This means you need to rest more to restock your limited energy supply.'   [The patient understands]

For the patient who has not yet come to terms with the situation:

'I think a few quiet days in bed are called for. If tomorrow or the next day you are feeling more energetic, of course you can get up but, for the moment, bed is the best place for you.'   [Not destroying hope, breaking bad news gently, giving the patient permission to let go]

For the spouse and close family:

'This weakness is normal. The cancer is like a parasite sapping all his energy.'   [The patient is not to blame. Also he is not odd or bad]

'I think the illness is beginning to win.'   [Time is short]

Although you may feel powerless in the face of rapidly approaching death, the patient is generally more realistic. He knows you cannot perform a miracle; he appreciates that time is limited.

- continue to visit

- quietly indicate that 'At this stage the important thing is to keep you as comfortable as possible'

- simplify medication, e.g. 'Now that your husband is not so well, he can probably manage without the heart tablets'

- arrange for medication to be given SL, PR or SC when the patient cannot swallow (*see* p.41)

- continue to inform the family of the changing situation:
    'He is very weak now, but he could still live for several days'
    'Although he seems better today, he is still very weak. He could quickly deteriorate and die in a day or so'

- control agitation even if it results in sedation (*see* p.308)

- listen to the nurses.

References

1   Gillon R (1994) Medical ethics: four principles plus attention to scope. *British Medical Journal.* **309**: 84–188.
2   Yaniv H (1994) Personal communication.

2 Pain relief

Pain

> 'Pain is what the patient says hurts.'

Pain is an unpleasant *sensory* and *emotional* experience associated with actual or potential tissue damage or described in terms of such damage. In other words, pain is a *somatopsychic* phenomenon. The perception of pain is therefore modulated by

* the patient's *mood*

* the patient's *morale*

* the *meaning* of the pain for the patient.

The meaning of persistent pain in advanced cancer is 'I am incurable, I am going to die'. Other factors affecting pain threshold are shown in Table 2.1. Because of the multidimensional nature of pain, it is often helpful to think in terms of total pain, encompassing the physical, psychological, social and spiritual aspects of suffering.

People with chronic pain generally do not look in pain because of the absence of autonomic concomitants (Table 2.2). In cancer, acute pain concomitants may be evident particularly if the pain is severe and of recent onset or paroxysmal.

Because of the implications for treatment, it is also important to distinguish between pain caused by stimulation of nerve endings (nociceptive pain) and pain caused by nerve dysfunction (neuropathic pain; Figure 2.1). Neuropathic pain is often only partially responsive to treatment with standard analgesics, including morphine and other opioids (*see* p.45). Thus, from a therapeutic

Table 2.1   Factors affecting pain threshold

Threshold lowered	Threshold raised
Discomfort	Relief of other symptoms
Insomnia	Sleep
Fatigue	Sympathy
Anxiety	Understanding
Fear	Companionship
Anger	Creative activity
Sadness	Relaxation
Depression	Reduction in anxiety
Boredom	Elevation of mood
Mental isolation	Analgesics
Social abandonment	Anxiolytics
	Antidepressants

Table 2.2   Temporal classification of pain

	Acute		Chronic	
Time course	Transient		Persistent	
Meaning to patient	Positive draws attention to injury or illness	Negative serves no useful purpose		Positive as patient obtains secondary gain
Concomitants	Fight or flight pupillary dilatation increased sweating tachypnoea tachycardia shunting of blood from viscera to muscles		Vegetative sleep disturbance anorexia decreased libido no pleasure in life constipation somatic pre-occupation personality change lethargy	

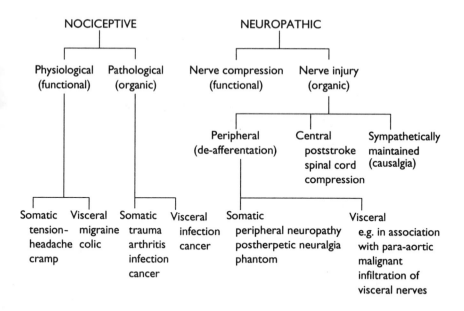

Figure 2.1 Classification of pain.

point of view, it is helpful to think of pain in terms of response to opioids (Table 2.3):

Opioid-responsive, i.e. pain relieved by opioids

Opioid-semiresponsive, i.e. pain relieved by the concurrent use of an opioid and an adjuvant drug (co-analgesic)

Opioid-resistant, i.e. pain not relieved by opioids.

Opioid resistance may be more apparent than real (Table 2.4). Painful muscle spasm (cramp) is a good example of true opioid-resistant pain. Cramp in various parts of the body is relatively common in cancer. It is often associated with bone pain which is exacerbated by movement. Anxiety is a potent exacerbating factor (Figure 2.2).

Myofascial pain is a specific form of cramp. It is associated with the presence of one or more hypersensitive points (trigger points) within muscle and/or the surrounding connective tissue together with muscle spasm, pain (often referred into neighbouring areas or the adjacent limb), tenderness, stiffness, limitation of movement, weakness and occasionally autonomic dysfunction. Myofascial trigger points occur most commonly in the pectoral girdle and neck (Figure 2.3).

Table 2.3 Types of pain and implications for treatment

Type of pain	Mechanism	Example	Response to opioids	Treatment
Nociceptive	Stimulation of nerve endings			
visceral		Hepatic capsule pain	+	Analgesics
somatic		Bone pain	+/–	Analgesics
muscle spasm			–	Muscle relaxant
Neuropathic				
nerve compression	Stimulation of nervi nervorum (?)		+/–	Analgesics; corticosteroid
nerve injury	Peripheral nerve injury (de-afferentation pain)	Neuroma or nerve infiltration (e.g. brachial or lumbosacral plexus)	(+)/–	Trial of opioid; trial of corticosteroid; tricyclic antidepressant; anticonvulsant; local anaesthetic congener; spinal analgesia; ketamine; TENS
	CNS injury	Spinal cord compression or poststroke pain		
sympathetically maintained	Abnormal sympathetic activity	Causalgia	–	Sympathetic nerve block

Table 2.4   Opioid-resistant cancer pain: clinical classification

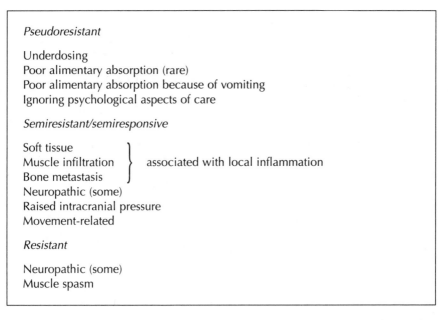

Pseudoresistant

Underdosing
Poor alimentary absorption (rare)
Poor alimentary absorption because of vomiting
Ignoring psychological aspects of care

Semiresistant/semiresponsive

Soft tissue ⎫
Muscle infiltration ⎬ associated with local inflammation
Bone metastasis ⎭
Neuropathic (some)
Raised intracranial pressure
Movement-related

Resistant

Neuropathic (some)
Muscle spasm

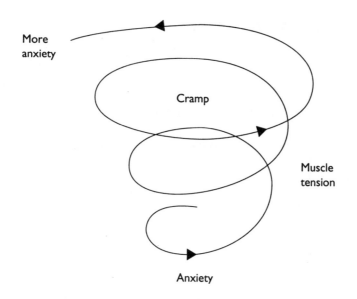

Figure 2.2   Relationship between anxiety and cramp.

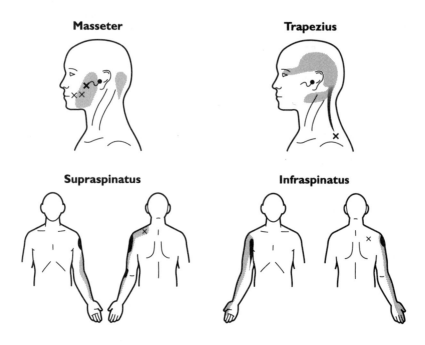

Figure 2.3   Selected trigger points and the associated patterns of local and referred myofascial pain.[1] Pain pattern ▬▬; Trigger area X.

Pain in advanced cancer

Pain and advanced cancer are not synonymous

- three quarters of patients experience pain
- one quarter of patients do not experience pain.

Multiple concurrent pains are common in those who have pain

- about one third has a single pain
- one third has two pains
- one third has three or more pains.[2]

Pain in cancer can be grouped into four causal categories

- caused by cancer itself (85% of patients)
- caused by treatment (17%)

- related to cancer and/or debility (9%)
- caused by a concurrent disorder (9%).[2]

In 15% of patients with advanced cancer and pain, none of the pain is caused by the cancer itself. Common individual causes are shown below (Table 2.5).

Table 2.5 Top 10 pains in patients with advanced cancer at Sobell House (*n* = 211)

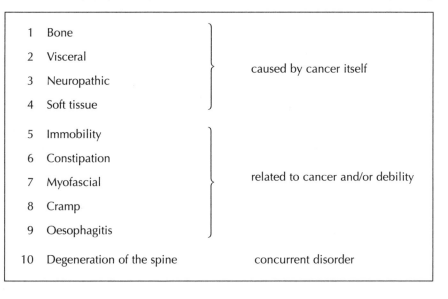

1	Bone	
2	Visceral	caused by cancer itself
3	Neuropathic	
4	Soft tissue	
5	Immobility	
6	Constipation	
7	Myofascial	related to cancer and/or debility
8	Cramp	
9	Oesophagitis	
10	Degeneration of the spine	concurrent disorder

Evaluation

Careful evaluation is necessary to prevent inappropriate treatment. Abdominal and/or rectal pain caused by constipation may be relieved by morphine but its use is clearly inappropriate. So too is the use of morphine for cramp and myofascial pain. Evaluation of pain in advanced cancer is primarily clinical and is based on *probability* and *pattern recognition*.

Neuropathic pain is described on page 43. A chart of neurodermatomes is helpful (Figure 2.4). The use of a body chart to record sites of pain is recommended (Figure 2.5).

When there is doubt, investigations should be undertaken urgently. These range from plain radiographs, through ultrasound and contrast radiography, to CT and MRI. Initial treatment should not be withheld, however, until these have been completed. Analgesics should be started (*see* p.24).

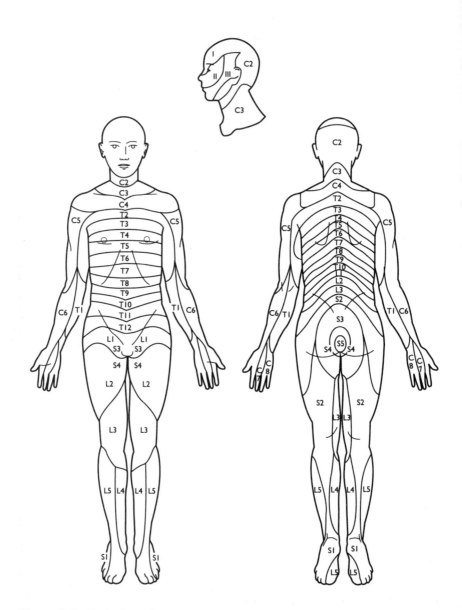

Figure 2.4 Body chart showing dermatomes, i.e. areas in which pain is experienced if the corresponding nerve is compressed or damaged.

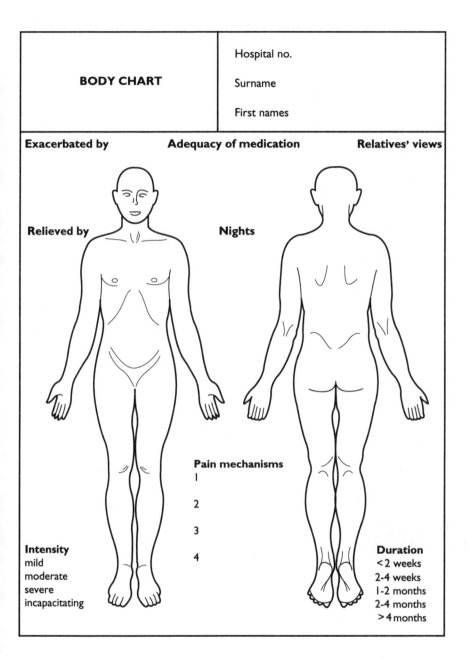

Figure 2.5 Overprinted body chart used at Sobell House for recording pain data.

Pain management

Pain relief often requires a broad-spectrum (i.e. multimodal) approach (Table 2.6). If anticancer treatment is recommended, analgesics should also be given until the treatment ameliorates the pain – which may take several weeks.

Table 2.6 Pain management in cancer

Examination	Psychological
	relaxation
To establish trust	cognitive-behavioural therapy
To confirm site	psychodynamic therapy
To identify cause	
	Interruption of pain pathways
Explanation to reduce psychological	
impact of pain	Local anaesthesia
	lidocaine
Modification of pathological process	bupivacaine
	Neurolysis
Radiation therapy	chemical (alcohol, phenol,
Hormone therapy	chlorocresol)
Chemotherapy	cold (cryotherapy)
Surgery	heat (thermocoagulation)
	Neurosurgery
Analgesics	cervical spinothalamic
	tractotomy (cordotomy)
Primary	
nonopioids	*Modification of way of life and*
opioids	*environment*
Secondary	
corticosteroids	Avoid pain-precipitating activities
antidepressants	Immobilization of the painful part
anticonvulsants	cervical collar
muscle relaxants	surgical corset
	slings
Nondrug methods	orthopaedic surgery
	Walking aid
Physical	Wheelchair
heat pads	Hoist
TENS	

Radiation should be considered whenever pain is caused by a bone metastasis or nerve compression. A single treatment with 6–10 Gy is often possible, particularly in peripheral sites.

Radiation gives partial or complete relief in > 80% of patients with bone pain.[3] Recalcification occurs in most of these. Radiation is also beneficial in several other situations (Table 2.7). It is generally inappropriate in patients with a very short life expectancy, i.e. < 2 weeks.

Table 2.7   Radiation therapy and symptom management

Bone pain	Malignant ulcer
	superficial
Compression	rectal
brachial plexus	
lumbosacral plexus	Blood loss
cauda equina	haemoptysis
spinal cord	haematuria
brain	vaginal
mediastinal obstruction	
porta hepatis	

The perception of pain requires both consciousness and attention. Pain is worse when it occupies a person's whole attention. Diversional activity does more than pass the time; it diminishes pain. Further, professional time spent exploring a patient's worries and fears is time well spent, and relates directly to pain management. If the patient is very anxious and/or depressed, it may take 2–4 weeks to achieve satisfactory relief.

Since the advent of spinal analgesia (see p.47), neurolytic and neurosurgical procedures have become almost obsolete in the UK. At many centres, coeliac axis plexus block with alcohol for epigastric visceral pain is the only neurolytic block still used. Internal fixation or the insertion of a prosthesis should be considered if a pathological fracture of a long bone occurs, or threatens. Such measures obviate the need for prolonged bed rest and pain is much reduced. The decision to treat surgically depends on the patient's general condition.

Some patients continue to experience pain on movement despite analgesics, other drugs, radiotherapy and nerve blocks. Here, the situation is often improved by suggesting modifications to the patient's way of life and environment. This is where the help of a physiotherapist and an occupational therapist is often invaluable.

It is generally best to aim at progressive pain relief

- relief at night
- relief at rest during the day
- relief on movement (not always completely possible).

Relief should be evaluated in relation to each pain. If there is severe anxiety and/or depression, it may take 3–4 weeks to achieve maximum benefit. Re-evaluation is a continuing necessity; old pains may get worse and new ones develop.

Principles of analgesic use

For pain caused by the cancer itself, drugs generally give adequate relief provided the right drug is administered in the right dose at the right time intervals.

By the mouth

The oral route is the preferred route for analgesics, including morphine and other strong opioids.

By the clock

Persistent pain requires preventive therapy. Analgesics should be given regularly and prophylactically. As needed medication is irrational and inhumane.

By the ladder

Use the 3-step analgesic ladder (Figure 2.6). If a drug fails to relieve, *move up the ladder*, do not move laterally in the same efficacy group.

Individual treatment

The right dose of an analgesic is the dose which relieves the pain.

Supervision

The response to treatment must be monitored to ensure that benefits of treatment are maximized and adverse effects minimized.

Adjuvant drugs

A laxative is almost always necessary with an opioid; about 50% of patients need an anti-emetic (Table 2.8).

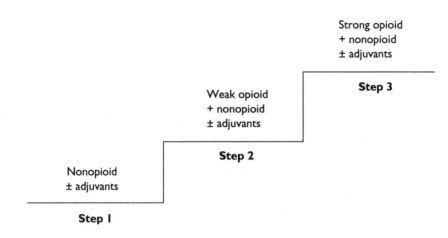

Figure 2.6   The World Health Organization 3-step analgesic ladder.[4]

Table 2.8   Adjuvant drugs for analgesic ladder

Control of adverse effects	*Secondary analgesics*
Laxative	Corticosteroid
Anti-emetic	Antidepressant
	Anticonvulsant
Psychotropic medication	Muscle relaxant
Night sedative	
Anxiolytic	
Antidepressant	

Nonopioids

The main nonopioids are

- aspirin

- other NSAIDs

- paracetamol/acetaminophen

Nonopioids are step 1 analgesics. Because of their anti-inflammatory effect, NSAIDs are particularly useful for metastatic bone and soft tissue pains. They should be used even when a strong opioid is also necessary.

In hot countries, NSAIDs are sometimes discouraged because of the risk of acute renal failure in hypovolaemic patients. Paracetamol is used instead.

Mode of action

Nonopioids inhibit prostaglandin (PG) synthesis by inhibiting the enzyme cyclo-oxygenase (COX). They do this to a variable extent in different tissues. Paracetamol inhibits PG synthesis in the brain but has no effect on PG synthesis in inflamed joints. Thus, although paracetamol is analgesic and antipyretic (like the NSAIDs), it is not anti-inflammatory in rheumatoid arthritis. Sulindac also shows selectivity; several studies (but not all) indicate less impact on renal PG synthesis.[5]

The relative benefits of the NSAIDs and paracetamol in painful bone metastases have yet to be determined. Likewise, the extent of the central analgesic effect of most NSAIDs is unknown.

COX exists in two forms. COX-1 is constitutive (i.e. present in all normal tissues), whereas COX-2 is normally undetectable in most tissues but massively induced by inflammation. By producing selective COX-2 inhibitors, it is hoped to reduce the gastric toxicity of NSAIDs (Figure 2.7).

Inhibition of PG synthesis does not account for the total analgesic effect of NSAIDs, although it appears to explain most of the adverse effects. In post-dental extraction pain, most weak COX inhibitors are significantly superior to aspirin and most strong inhibitors inferior. Ketorolac is an example of a weak COX inhibitor which is superior to aspirin and most other NSAIDs in terms of analgesic efficacy.

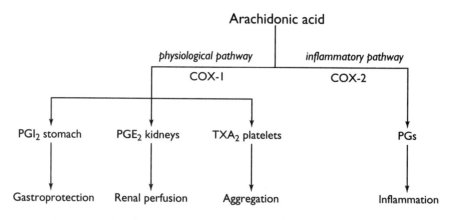

Figure 2.7   The functions of cyclo-oxygenase (COX).
PG = prostaglandin; TX = thromboxane.

Nonopioids and platelet function

- aspirin causes *irreversible* impairment of platelet function (with pro-longation of bleeding time) by inactivating platelet COX permanently by acetylation

- most other NSAIDs cause reversible impairment of platelet function

- *nonacetylated salicylates* have no effect on platelet function at normal therapeutic doses:
    choline magnesium salicylate
    diflunisal
    salsalate

- preferential COX-2 inhibitors do not affect platelet function at recom-mended doses: ↘
    meloxicam[6]
    nimesulide (not available in UK).[7]

Common adverse effects and interactions

- gastric erosions, peptic ulcers, haemorrhage:
    more with cheap standard aspirin tablets because of coarse granular
        nature
    less with dispersible and enteric-coated aspirin, similar to other
        NSAIDs
    ibuprofen (available 'over the counter') is least toxic in this respect

- many NSAIDs and paracetamol induce bronchospasm in susceptible patients; choline salicylate, choline magnesium trisalicylate, azapropazone, nimesulide and benzydamine do not

- aspirin may cause tinnitus and deafness, particularly in hypo-albuminaemic patients

- all NSAIDs cause salt and water retention which may result in ankle oedema. In consequence, they *antagonize* the action of diuretics to a variable extent

- aspirin *potentiates* oral hypoglycaemic agents

- aspirin *antagonizes* uricosuric agents

- NSAIDs can cause renal failure (acute or acute-on-chronic), particularly in patients with hypovolaemia from any cause, e.g. diuretics, fever, dehydration, vomiting, diarrhoea, haemorrhage, surgery. Also in other situations in which there are elevated plasma concentrations of vasoconstrictor substances such as angiotensin-II, norepinephrine and vasopressin, e.g. in heart failure, cirrhosis and nephrotic syndrome. The inhibition of renal PG production by a NSAID means that the protective vasodilatory mechanism for safeguarding renal blood flow is not able to function effectively[8]

- NSAIDs may also cause interstitial nephritis (+/– nephrotic syndrome or +/– papillary necrosis); this is sporadic and unpredictable.

Distinguishing features of paracetamol

- it can be taken by most patients who are hypersensitive to aspirin; cross-sensitivity occurs in only 25%

- it does not injure the gastric mucosa

- it is well tolerated by patients with peptic ulcers

- it does not affect plasma uric acid concentration

- it has no effect on platelet function

- liquid preparations are stable

- adverse effects are uncommon.

The main drawback with paracetamol is the frequency of administration (q4h–q6h). Because NSAIDs are mainly peripheral in action and paracetamol central, the two can be used together with an additive effect.

Choice of NSAID

This depends on several factors, e.g. availability, fashion, cost, frequency of administration, individual toxicity and response. Typical regimens include:

Ibuprofen	400–600 mg q.d.s.
Flurbiprofen	50–100 mg b.d.
Naproxen	250–500 mg b.d.
Diflunisal	250–500 mg b.d.
Diclofenac m/r	150–200 mg o.d.
Benorylate suspension	5–10 ml b.d.

Relative toxicity is shown in Table 2.9.

Table 2.9   Risk of NSAID-related gastroduodenal toxicity

Lowest	Intermediate	Highest
Ibuprofen	Diclofenac	Azapropazone
Meloxicam	Diflunisal	Ketorolac
Nimesulide	Flurbiprofen	
	Indometacin	
	Ketoprofen	
	Naproxen	
	Piroxicam	

Diclofenac 150 mg and ketorolac 30–60 mg are used by SC infusion at some centres. Tenoxicam 20 mg SC/IM o.d. is a useful alternative and may obviate the need for a second syringe driver in a patient requiring multiple parenteral drugs (*see* p.42).

Piroxicam 20 mg, given as Feldene Melt tablets, is another option; this dissolves rapidly and completely if placed on the tongue or in the mouth. Absorption is gastro-intestinal, however, which means that Feldene Melt tablets should not be used in patients who cannot swallow their saliva.

Weak opioids

Weak opioids in combination with nonopioids are step 2 analgesics (Table 2.10). A weak opioid is as effective as a small dose of morphine. This means that step 2 is pharmacologically unnecessary. In many countries, however, it is much easier to obtain and supply a weak opioid preparation.

Table 2.10   Commonly used weak opioid compound preparations (UK)

| Generic name | | Drug content | |
		Weak opioid	Nonopioid
Co-codaprin	8/400	Codeine 8 mg	Aspirin 400 mg
Co-codamol	8/500	Codeine 8 mg	Paracetamol 500 mg
Co-codamol	30/500	Codeine 30 mg	Paracetamol 500 mg
Co-dydramol	10/500	Dihydrocodeine 10 mg	Paracetamol 500 mg
Co-proxamol	32.5/325	Dextropropoxyphene hydrochloride 32.5 mg	Paracetamol 325 mg

Codeine is a prodrug of morphine.[9] It is about 1/10 as potent as morphine. *About 10% of the population cannot convert codeine to morphine.* The typical dose range for codeine is 30–60 mg q4h. Dihydrocodeine is generally used instead in the UK.

Tramadol

Tramadol is an alternative opioid for both step 2 and the lower end of step 3. Its exact relative potency with oral codeine and oral morphine in cancer patients is still debatable. By injection, it is 1/10 as potent as mophine. In Table 2.11 (*see* p.35), it is regarded as double strength codeine, i.e. 1/5 strength morphine. This difference relates to the high oral bio-availability of tramadol (about 70%).

Tramadol has a dual mechanism of analgesic action, part opioid and part a presynaptic re-uptake blocker of mono-amines (like a tricyclic antidepressant; *see* p.50). It does not have anticholinergic or antidepressant properties. The dual analgesic action is synergistic. Adverse opioid effects are significantly less than with codeine and morphine.

There is circumstantial evidence that tramadol lowers seizure threshold. Patients with a history of epilepsy should generally *not* be prescribed tramadol. Tramadol should be used with caution in patients taking other medication which lowers seizure threshold, notably tricyclic antidepressants and SSRIs.

Strong opioids

These are step 3 analgesics. As in step 2, a nonopioid should normally be given concurrently.

Morphine and other strong opioids exist to be given, not merely to be withheld. Their use is dictated by therapeutic need, not by brevity of prognosis.

Morphine does not cause clinically important respiratory depression in cancer patients in pain. This is because *pain is a physiological antagonist to the central depressant effects of morphine.* Thus, it is extremely rare to need to use naloxone, a specific opioid antagonist, in palliative care (*see* p.40). Further, in contrast to postoperative patients, cancer patients with pain

- have generally been receiving a weak opioid for some time, i.e. are not opioid naive
- take medication by mouth (slower absorption, lower peak concentration)

- titrate the dose upwards step by step (less likelihood of an excessive dose being given).

The relationship of the therapeutic dose to the lethal dose of morphine (the therapeutic ratio) is greater than commonly supposed. Patients who take a double dose of morphine at bedtime are no more likely to die during the night than those who do not.[10]

Morphine is metabolized mainly to morphine-3-glucuronide and morphine-6-glucuronide. The former is inactive, whereas the latter is *more* potent as an analgesic than morphine itself. Both glucuronides cumulate in renal failure. This results in a prolonged duration of action for morphine, with a danger of severe sedation and subsequent respiratory depression if the dose and/or frequency of administration are not reduced.

Tolerance to morphine is not a practical problem. Psychological dependence (addiction) does not occur if morphine is used correctly. Physical dependence does not prevent a reduction in the dose of morphine if the patient's pain ameliorates, e.g. as a result of radiotherapy or a nerve block.

Morphine is not the panacea for cancer pain. Its use does not guarantee success, particularly if the psychosocial aspects of care are ignored.

The next four sections form a synopsis of Chapter 3 (*see* p.60).

Oral morphine

From a global perspective, morphine by mouth is the strong opioid of choice for cancer pain. It is administered as tablets (10 mg, 20 mg) or in aqueous solution (e.g. 2 mg in 1 ml). An increasing range of m/r preparations is available – tablets, capsules, suspensions. Most are administered b.d., some o.d.

If the patient was previously receiving a weak opioid, begin with 10 mg q4h (or m/r 30 mg q12h). With frail elderly patients, consider starting on 5 mg q4h in order to reduce initial drowsiness, confusion and unsteadiness.

If changing from an alternative strong opioid (e.g. buprenorphine, levorphanol, methadone), a much higher dose of morphine may be needed (*see* p.35).

Adjust the dose upwards after 24 h if the pain is not 90% relieved (e.g. 5 → 10 mg, 10 → 15 mg, 20 → 30 mg). Two thirds of patients never need more than 30 mg q4h (or m/r morphine 100 mg q12h). The rest need up to 200 mg q4h (or m/r morphine 600 mg q12h) and occasionally more.

Additional rescue doses of morphine should be prescribed for breakthrough pain. Instructions must be clear: extra morphine does not mean that the next dose of regular morphine is omitted.

If extra morphine is requested several times a day, the regular dose should be adjusted upwards.

With ordinary tablets or solution, a double dose at bedtime generally enables a patient to go through the night without waking in pain.

Morphine should generally be given together with a nonopioid.

Supply an anti-emetic for regular use should nausea or vomiting develop, e.g. haloperidol 1.5 mg stat and nocte.

Prescribe laxatives, e.g. co-danthrusate or senna + docusate. Adjust dose according to response. Suppositories and enemas continue to be necessary in about one third of patients. *Constipation may be more difficult to manage than the pain.*

Warn patients about the possibility of initial drowsiness.

Write out the drug regimen in detail with times, names of drugs and amount to be taken (*see* pp 8, 9); arrange for follow-up.

If swallowing is difficult or vomiting persists, morphine may be given PR by suppository (same dose as PO). Alternatively, give half of the oral dose of morphine by SC injection or one third of the dose as SC diamorphine.

Improving drug compliance

Because many wards have only four drug rounds a day (0600, 1200, 1800 and 2200 h), special provision has to be made to enable a patient to receive morphine q4h. In practice, the interval between the first drug round (0600 h) and the last (2200 h) is generally less than 16 h, and it is not uncommon to see a series of entries such as:

0725, 1125, 1550, 2130 h *or*

0725, 1125, 1525, 1925, 2350 h

In the first example, it proved impossible to give the third dose on time and the fourth has been delayed partly for convenience and partly to 'help you have a better night'. In the second example, the nurses have coped with a highly individual regimen until bedtime, but then 'Here is your night sedative, Mr Smith. You cannot have your morphine yet, it's not due. We'll bring it later'.

The patient either fails to get to sleep because of worry about the pain returning or complains bitterly when woken from a deep sleep by a nurse an hour or so later. In both instances, the comfort (and sleep) of the patient is put in jeopardy by a pharisaical attitude to the concept of 'every four hours'.

It is often necessary to catch up at some stage in the day. Catching up is best done at 1000 h. If 'time slippage' occurs later in the day, catching up should be repeated, preferably at the next administration and certainly at 2200 h.

The interval between the early morning dose and the 1000 h dose is generally less than 4 h, occasionally less than 3 h. The nurses should be advised specifically on this point.

When catching up is practised, it is much easier for the nurses to administer medication q4h. In fact, the only administration additional to the routine drug rounds is 1000 h. This is a time when the maximum number of nurses are available, and when Controlled Drug book-keeping is easiest to complete.

Check daily to ensure that all the prescribed doses have been given.

The availability of m/r tablets has simplified considerably the use of morphine on general wards.

Diamorphine

Diamorphine hydrochloride (di-acetylmorphine, heroin) is available for medicinal use only in the UK and Canada. It is much more soluble than morphine sulphate/hydrochloride and is used in the UK instead of morphine when injections are necessary because large amounts can be given in very small volumes.

By injection, diamorphine is twice as potent as morphine. By this route, its initial effects are mediated by the primary metabolite, mono-acetylmorphine.

Because of rapid de-acetylation, diamorphine by mouth is merely a prodrug for morphine. Possibly because of better absorption (it is highly lipid-soluble), it is slightly more potent than morphine by this route.

Converting from morphine to diamorphine or changing routes

The following conversion ratios are approximate and should be regarded only as a general guide[11]

* oral morphine to SC morphine, halve the oral dose
* oral morphine to IV morphine, give one third of the oral dose

- oral morphine to SC diamorphine, give one third of the oral dose
- oral diamorphine to SC diamorphine, halve the oral dose.

When changing from either oral diamorphine or oral morphine to m/r morphine, convert 1 mg for 1 mg and adjust as necessary.

There are no generic m/r morphine tablets. Because of differing pharmacokinetic profiles, it is best to keep individual patients on the same brand.

Alternative strong opioids

There are multiple opioid receptor subtypes in many areas of the CNS, including the dorsal horn of the spinal cord. Mu, kappa and delta opioid receptors are all involved in analgesia. Opioids differ from each other in terms of intrinsic activity and receptor site affinity. This property can be utilized in patients who are intolerant of morphine (mainly a mu agonist) by converting, for example, to methadone (a mixed mu and delta agonist).

When converting from an alternative strong opioid to oral morphine, the initial dose depends on the relative potency of the two drugs (Table 2.11). Table 2.11 should also be used to determine an appropriate starting dose of an alternative opioid in someone intolerant of morphine (e.g. marked dysphoria and/or sedation, hallucinations, nausea and vomiting, pruritus, which fail to respond to appropriate measures; *see* p.78).

Pethidine and dextromoramide have little place in cancer pain management because of short durations of action. Some centres use dextromoramide for breakthrough pain in patients taking regular morphine, or as prophylactic additional analgesia before a painful dressing or other procedure. This is because of its rapid onset of action. Generally, patients obtain satisfactory relief from an additional dose of morphine or by timing the procedure for 1 h after a regular dose.

Pentazocine should not be used; it is a weak opioid by mouth and often causes psychotomimetic effects (dysphoria, depersonalization, frightening dreams, hallucinations).

Phenazocine

Phenazocine is available in the UK as a scored 5 mg tablet which can be taken either PO or SL. It has been used at some centres for many years as a convenient alternative strong opioid in patients intolerant of morphine. Each

Table 2.11   Approximate oral analgesic equivalence to morphine[a]

Analgesic	Potency ratio with morphine	Duration of action (h)[b]
Codeine } Dihydrocodeine	1/10	3–5
Pethidine (meperidine USA)	1/8	2–3
Tramadol	1/5[c]	5–6
Dipipanone (in Diconal UK)	1/2	3–5
Papaveretum	2/3[d]	3–5
Oxycodone	1.5–2[c]	5–6
Dextromoramide	[2][e]	2–3
Levorphanol	5	6–8
Phenazocine	5	6–8
Methadone	5–10[f]	8–12
Hydromorphone	7.5	3–5
Buprenorphine (*sublingual*)	60	6–8
Fentanyl (*transdermal*)	150	72

a   multiply dose of opioid by its potency ratio to determine the equivalent dose of morphine sulphate

b   dependent in part on severity of pain and on dose; often longer lasting in very elderly and those with renal dysfunction

c   tramadol and oxycodone are both relatively more potent by mouth because of high bio-availability; parenteral potency ratios with morphine are 1/10 and 3/4 respectively

d   papaveretum (strong opium) is standardized to contain 50% morphine base; potency expressed in relation to morphine sulphate

e   dextromoramide: a single 5 mg dose is equivalent to morphine 15 mg in terms of peak effect but is shorter acting; overall potency ratio adjusted accordingly

f   methadone: by injection, a single 5 mg dose is equivalent to morphine 7.5 mg. However, its long plasma halflife and its broad-spectrum receptor affinity result in a much higher than expected potency ratio when given repeatedly.[12]

5 mg tablet is equivalent to about 25 mg of morphine. It often needs to be given only q6h. Individual doses of up to 20 mg have been used. Its receptor site affinities have not been determined but it is probably mainly a mu agonist.

Methadone

Methadone is a mixed mu and delta opioid agonist and a NMDA-receptor antagonist.[13] Some patients with nociceptive pain who obtain only poor relief with morphine but severe adverse effects (drowsiness, delirium, nausea and vomiting) obtain good relief with relatively low doses of methadone with few or no adverse effects.

Methadone is also useful in patients with renal failure who develop excessive drowsiness and/or delirium with morphine because of cumulation of morphine-6-glucuronide. Methadone does not have a comparable active metabolite and its effects are not altered in renal failure.

The plasma halflife of methadone ranges from 8–80 h and is affected by changes in urinary pH. Cumulation is a potential problem for most patients. Dose titration is therefore different from morphine. For 2–3 days patients are advised to take a dose *q3h as needed*; after this most patients can be converted to either a b.d. or t.d.s. regimen.

Oxycodone

Oxycodone is a mu agonist with similar properties to morphine.[14,15] Although oxycodone has no clinically important active metabolites, the maximum plasma concentration increases by 50% in renal failure causing more sedation.[16] It has a plasma halflife of about 3.5 h, which is prolonged by about 1 h in renal failure. Parenterally it is about 3/4 as potent as morphine.[16] However, oral bioavailability is 2/3 or more, compared with about 1/3 for morphine. This means that oxycodone by mouth is about 1.5–2 times more potent than oral morphine.[17,18] Oxycodone is generally given q4h but could possibly be given q6h in some patients. An oral preparation is not yet available in the UK.

Hydromorphone

Hydromorphone is an analogue of morphine with similar pharmacokinetic and pharmacodynamic properties. By mouth and by injection it is about 7.5 times more potent than morphine.[19] As with morphine, there is wide interpatient variation in bio-availability.

Hydromorphone is available in many countries in a range of preparations for oral, rectal and parenteral administration. In the UK, hydromorphone is available as ordinary capsules (1.3 and 2.6 mg = morphine 10 and 20 mg) and m/r capsules (2, 4, 8, 16, 24 mg = m/r morphine 15, 30, 60, 120, 180 mg). In some countries (but *not* the UK), hydromorphone is available in high potency ampoules containing 10 mg/ml and 20 mg/ml to facilitate use in continuous SC infusions. Hydromorphone provides useful analgesia for about 4 h.

Fentanyl

Fentanyl, like morphine, is mainly a strong mu agonist. It is widely used as a peri-operative analgesic. Transdermal patches (Durogesic) are available for cancer pain management. These deliver 25, 50, 75 or 100 mcg/h over 3 days. Patients who have not previously taken morphine or other strong opioids should always be started on the lowest dose, i.e. 25 mcg/h (Table 2.12).

Table 2.12   Converting oral morphine sulphate to transdermal fentanyl[20]

Oral morphine (mg q4h)	Oral morphine (mg/day)	Transdermal fentanyl delivery rate (mcg/h)
5–20	30–120	25
25–35	150–210	50
40–50	240–300	75
55–65	330–390	100
70–80	420–480	125
85–95	510–570	150

Steady-state plasma concentrations of fentanyl are achieved after 36–48 h.[21] Time to reach a minimal effective plasma concentration ranges from 3–23 h.[21] After removal of a patch, the elimination plasma halflife is almost 24 h,[22] compared with 3–4 h after a single IV injection.[23] Rescue medication will be necessary particularly during the first 24 h.

In some patients the potency ratio for oral morphine and transdermal fentanyl may be only half that recommended by the manufacturer, i.e. 70 rather than 150.[24] Accordingly, some centres use a conversion factor of 100 to determine the initial patch strength.[24]

If effective analgesia does not last for 3 days, the correct response is to increase the patch strength. Even so, a few patients do best if the patch is changed every 2 days. High fever and exposure of transdermal patches to external heat sources (e.g. heat pads, electric blankets) may increase the rate of delivery of fentanyl.

Transdermal fentanyl is less constipating than morphine.[25] Thus, when converting from morphine to fentanyl, the dose of laxative should be halved and subsequently adjusted according to need (Figure 2.8). Some patients experience abdominal withdrawal symptoms when changed from morphine PO to transdermal fentanyl despite satisfactory pain relief, i.e. colic, diarrhoea and nausea together with sweating and restlessness. These symptoms are easily treatable by using rescue doses of morphine until they resolve after a few days.

Transdermal fentanyl can be continued until the death of the patient, and the dose varied as necessary. Rescue medication will continue to be ordinary morphine tablets or solution (or an alternative 'immediate-release' strong opioid preparation). When a patient is no longer able to swallow oral medication, most essential drugs tend to be given PR or parenterally, e.g. by continuous SC infusion. Although there is no need to change transdermal fentanyl, it is important to give adequate rescue doses of diamorphine (in the UK) or of an alternative strong opioid (Box 2A).

Box 2.A   Parenteral rescue medication for patients receiving transdermal fentanyl

Divide the delivery rate ('patch size') of transdermal fentanyl (mcg/h)

- by 3 and give as SC morphine (mg)
- by 5 and give as SC diamorphine (mg)
- by 15 and give as SC hydromorphone (mg)

Buprenorphine

Buprenorphine is a potent partial mu agonist, kappa antagonist and delta agonist. It is an alternative to oral morphine in the low to middle part of morphine's dose range.

In low doses, buprenorphine and morphine are additive in their effects; at very high doses, antagonism by buprenorphine may occur. There is no need, however, to prescribe both; use one or the other.

Buprenorphine is available as a *sublingual* tablet; ingestion reduces bioavailability. It needs to be given only q8h. More frequent administration

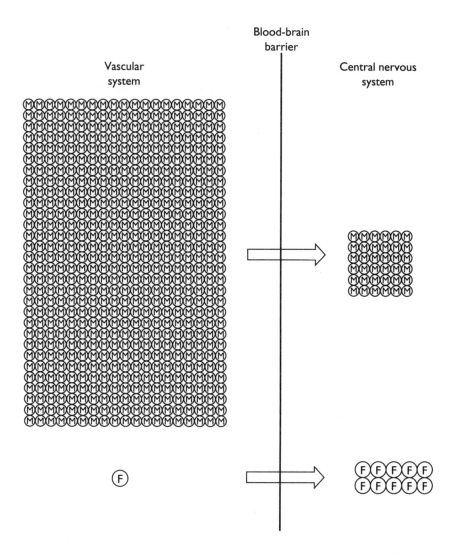

Figure 2.8 Distribution of equipotent doses of morphine and fentanyl in the vascular and central nervous systems based on animal data.[26] Converting from oral or parenteral morphine to transdermal or parenteral fentanyl will result in a massive decrease in opioid molecules outside the CNS. This will result in less constipation and could, in physically dependent subjects, precipitate peripherally-mediated withdrawal symptoms. Further, because opioids within the brain have an anti-emetic effect (in contrast to opioids in the vascular system), it can be predicted that fentanyl will cause less nausea and vomiting than morphine.

makes life unnecessarily harder for a hard-pressed patient. With daily doses of over 3 mg, patients may prefer to take fewer tablets q6h.

It is generally considered that there is an analgesic ceiling at a daily dose of 3–5 mg; equivalent to 180–300 mg of oral morphine/24 h. In some countries, 1.6 mg is regarded as the ceiling daily dose. Whether this represents genetic differences or local custom is not clear.

Buprenorphine is not an alternative to codeine or other weak opioid. Like morphine, it should be used when a weak opioid has failed. Assuming the previous regular use of a weak opioid, patients should commence on 200 mcg q8h with the advice that, 'If it is not more effective than your previous tablets take a further 200 mcg after 1 h, and 400 mcg q8h after that.'

When changing to morphine, multiply the total daily dose of buprenorphine by 60. If the pain was previously poorly relieved, multiply by 100. Adverse effects, e.g. nausea, vomiting, constipation, drowsiness, need to be monitored as with morphine.

Naloxone

The BNF contains two entries for naloxone. One relates to overdosage by addicts and recommends *0.8–2 mg* IV every 2–3 min up to a total of 10 mg if necessary, with the possibility of an ongoing IV infusion.

The other relates to reversal of respiratory depression caused by the medicinal use of opioids. In this circumstance, *100–200 mcg* IV should be given, with increments of *100 mcg* every 2 min until respiratory function is satisfactory. Further doses should be given after 1–2 h by IM injection if there is concern that further absorption of the opioid will result in delayed respiratory depression. Even lower doses have been recommended by others (Box 2.B).

It is important *not* to measure the response by level of consciousness because total antagonism will cause a return of severe pain with hyperalgesia and, if physically dependent, severe physical withdrawal symptoms and agitation. For respiratory depression with epidural morphine, however, it is safe to give 0.4 mg. In this circumstance, naloxone reverses respiratory depression without reversing analgesia.[27]

Box 2.B Naloxone for iatrogenic opioid overdose (based on the recommendations of the American Pain Society)[28]

If respiratory rate $\geq$ 8/min and patient not cyanosed, adopt a policy of 'wait and see'.

If life-threatening respiratory depression, dilute a standard ampoule containing naloxone 400 mcg/1 ml to 10 ml with saline for injection.

Administer 0.5 ml (20 mcg) IV every 2 min until the patient's respiratory status is satisfactory.

Further boluses may be necessary every 30–60 min because naloxone is shorter acting than morphine (and other opioids).

Continuous subcutaneous infusions

When oral administration is no longer feasible, continuous SC infusion of morphine sulphate, diamorphine hydrochloride or hydromorphone obviates the need for injections q4h. Particularly for ambulant patients, however, transdermal fentanyl provides a more convenient alternative (*see* p.37).

Indications for SC infusions

- intractable vomiting
- severe dysphagia
- patient too weak to swallow oral drugs
- poor alimentary absorption (rare).

Advantages

- constant analgesia (no peaks or troughs)
- usually reloaded once in 24 h
- comfort and confidence (no repeated injections)
- does not limit mobility
- permits better control of nausea and vomiting.

Choice of drugs

Because most patients receive several drugs in one syringe, miscibility and stability must be considered. The BNF advises that the following can be mixed with diamorphine

- cyclizine

- dexamethasone

- haloperidol

- hyoscine butylbromide

- hyoscine hydrobromide

- levomepromazine

- metoclopramide

- midazolam.

The following limitations should be noted

- cyclizine may precipitate at concentrations above 20 mg/ml, or in the presence of saline, or as the concentration of diamorphine relative to cyclizine increases; mixtures of diamorphine and cyclizine are also liable to precipitate after 24 h

- special care is needed to avoid precipitation of dexamethasone, i.e. warm the syringe by holding it in closed hand before adding dexamethasone

- mixtures of haloperidol and diamorphine are liable to precipitate after 24 h if haloperidol concentration is above 2 mg/ml

- occasionally metoclopramide may become discoloured; such solutions should be discarded

- cyclizine generally precipitates if mixed with metoclopramide, but they should not be used together because anticholinergic drugs block the intestinal action of metoclopramide

- diclofenac and ketorolac mix with diamorphine, provided the drugs are drawn up in saline; they do not mix with other drugs

- phenobarbital is miscible only with diamorphine and hyoscine

- chlorpromazine can be given SC but tends to cause local SC inflammation

- prochlorperazine and diazepam are too irritant for SC infusion.

Choice of infusion sites

- upper chest (intercostal plane)
- upper arm (outer aspect)
- abdomen
- thighs.

If the infusion causes painful local inflammation, consider

- changing the needle site prophylactically, e.g. daily
- reducing the quantity of the irritant drug
- changing to an alternative drug, e.g. cyclizine to hyoscine
- giving the irritant drug IM or PR
- adding hydrocortisone sodium succinate 25–50 mg to the syringe
- adding hyaluronidase 1500 units to the syringe.

Neuropathic pain

Description

Neuropathic pain is pain associated with neuropathy, i.e. nerve compression and nerve injury (somatic, visceral, sympathetic) or CNS lesions. Pain in an area of abnormal or absent sensation is always neuropathic.

Pathogenesis

There are many causes of neuropathic pain in cancer (Table 2.13). Such pain stems from three different mechanisms.

Nerve compression

For example, nerve root compression caused by a collapsed vertebra. It manifests as mild, moderate or severe aching pain in a neurodermatomal distribution.

Table 2.13　Causes of neuropathic pain in advanced cancer

Caused by cancer	*Related to cancer and/or debility*
Nerve compression/infiltration Plexopathy Spinal cord compression Thalamic tumour	Postherpetic neuralgia
Caused by treatment	*Concurrent causes*
Postoperative incisional pain Phantom limb pain Chemotherapy (peripheral neuropathy) Radiation (brachial plexopathy)	Diabetic neuropathy Poststroke pain

Nerve injury

For example, brachial and lumbosacral plexus infiltration by cancer. This may evolve from earlier nerve compression.

Nerve injury causes pain as a result of

- neuronal hyperexcitability:
  spontaneous activity
  mechanical sensitivity
  α-adrenergic sensitivity

- a cascade of neurochemical and physiological changes in the CNS, particularly in the dorsal horn of the spinal cord.

Nerve injury does not always lead to pain, e.g. postherpetic neuralgia is rare in young people. Further, with identical lesions, only a minority develop pain. A genetic factor has been postulated.

Sympathetically maintained pain

This is an uncommon form of neuropathic pain, related to sympathetic nerve trauma at operation or 'irritation' by a tumour. It is similar to somatic nerve injury pain but has an arterial distribution instead of a neurodermatomal one. It differs also in its response to treatment.

Clinical features of nerve injury pain

Distribution

Neurodermatomal, if peripheral lesion.

Quality

Superficial burning/stinging pain, particularly if peripheral lesion; +/– spontaneous stabbing/shooting pain. There may also be a deep aching component.

Concomitants

- often receiving morphine with little effect; and exhausted by insomnia
- allodynia (light touch exacerbates pain); unable to bear clothing against affected area
- sensory deficit, e.g. numbness
- sometimes a sympathetic component manifests as cutaneous vasodilation, increased skin temperature, changes in sweating pattern.

Management

Explanation

Nerve compression pain
'Needs cortisone as well as painkillers.'

Nerve injury pain
'Often does not respond well to painkillers, e.g. aspirin and morphine.'
'Need to start a different type of painkiller.'
'First step is to get a good night's sleep.'

Drugs of choice

Nerve compression pain
A combination of morphine and a corticosteroid, e.g. dexamethasone 4–8 mg o.d., is often effective (Figure 2.9).

Nerve injury pain
This is often relatively resistant to morphine and corticosteroids. When this is so, it is necessary to use one or more secondary analgesics, i.e. drugs not marketed primarily as analgesics but of proven value in relieving nerve injury pain (Figure 2.10).

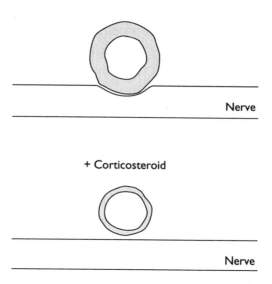

+ Corticosteroid

Figure 2.9   Possible mechanism of action of corticosteroids in relief of nerve compression pain. Total tumour mass = neoplasm + surrounding inflammation. General anti-inflammatory effect of corticosteroid reduces total tumour mass resulting in reduction of pain.

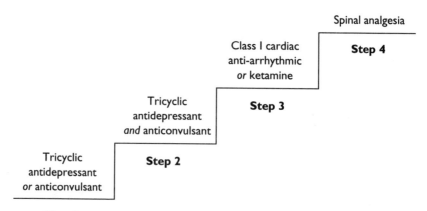

Figure 2.10   A 4-step analgesic ladder for nerve injury pain; used either alone or in conjunction with the WHO 3-step ladder, depending on circumstances.

Many centres use a tricyclic antidepressant for superficial burning pain and allodynia, and use an anticonvulsant for spontaneous stabbing/shooting pain. Controlled studies indicate, however, that both are equally effective in both types of pain.[29,30] An anticonvulsant such as sodium valproate may act quicker than a tricyclic antidepressant. Note

- some centres use a class 1 cardiac anti-arrhythmic, e.g. flecainide or mexiletine as the drug of choice for nerve injury pain, i.e. it is used as step 1. These are chemically related to local anaesthetics

- ketamine (a dissociative anaesthetic and NMDA receptor antagonist) is given in subanaesthetic doses (Box 2.C)

- some centres move straight from step 2 to step 4 (Figure 2.11); spinal analgesia includes both epidural and intrathecal routes

- nerve injury pain is more responsive to spinal morphine than morphine by conventional routes. (Spinal analgesia is also used occasionally in patients with nociceptive pain who experience intolerable adverse effects with PO or SC morphine)

- some patients benefit from TENS

- the putative mechanisms of secondary analgesics are shown in Figure 2.12.

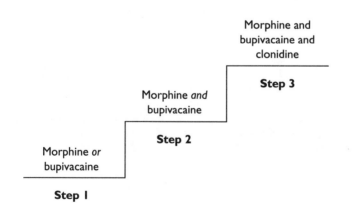

Figure 2.11   A 3-step ladder for spinal analgesia. In the concentrations generally used, bupivacaine acts as a local analgesic without significant sensory or motor effects; its main impact is probably on neuropathic pain. Clonidine potentiates the effects of spinal morphine and bupivacaine, either separately or together. In the UK, diamorphine is often substituted for morphine.

Box 2.C   Ketamine in cancer pain management

A dissociative anaesthetic used mainly as an IV anaesthetic induction agent.

Its analgesic action is mediated mainly at spinal level where it acts as a NMDA receptor antagonist. Activation of the NMDA receptor-channel complex occurs in dorsal horn sensitization – a circumstance in which opioids are relatively ineffective.[31]

Used occasionally in palliative care for intractable pain, particularly neuropathic and inflammatory.[32] Can be administered by PO, SC, IM, IV, ED and IT routes and has a plasma halflife of about 3 h. The main metabolite, norketamine, is about 1/3 as potent as the parent compound.

Typical starting doses are ketamine 100–200 mg/24 h by continuous SC infusion, increasing by 100 mg/24 h to 600 mg/24 h. Higher doses have been used, up to 2.4 g/24 h.[33] The patient may feel sedated and/or dysphoric. The dose of the previously prescribed morphine is progressively reduced as pain relief improves.

Causes tachycardia and intracranial hypertension and should generally be avoided in patients with intracranial tumours and/or a history of epilepsy.

Has a propensity to cause hallucinations, particularly as the effects of a bolus dose wear off. Traditionally, diazepam or midazolam has been used to relieve these, in preference to an antipsychotic.

Experience with ketamine in palliative care is limited and no controlled data are available. It does not work every time; this could be caused by a failure to escalate the dose above 600 mg/24 h.

Some centres use ketamine PO (taken from ampoules) 10–200 mg q.d.s.–q4h and report success.[34] Given a maximum oral bio-availability of 20%, these doses are equivalent to 2–40 mg SC.

Is used less often in centres where methadone is substituted for morphine if the dose escalates to multigramme levels (see p.36) and in centres where spinal analgesia is readily available.

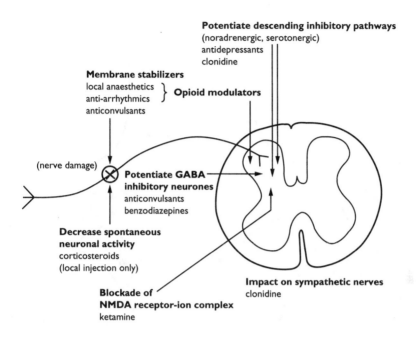

Figure 2.12 Impact of secondary analgesics on peripheral nerves and the dorsal horn of the spinal cord.

Sympathetically maintained pain

This responds to sympathetic nerve blocks (stellate ganglion or lumbar sympathetic chain); it does not respond to secondary analgesics.

Therapeutic guidelines

Tricyclic antidepressant

e.g. amitriptyline 25–75 mg nocte

The rate of increase in dose depends on pain intensity and extent of supervision. Relief may not occur for 4–5 days and is uncommon with only 25 mg. In cancer-related neuropathic pain, prescribe an anticonvulsant concurrently if amitriptyline 50 mg does not achieve satisfactory relief. Adverse effects are a common limiting factor. The mechanism of analgesic action is principally by potentiation of descending inhibitory pathways (Figure 2.13).

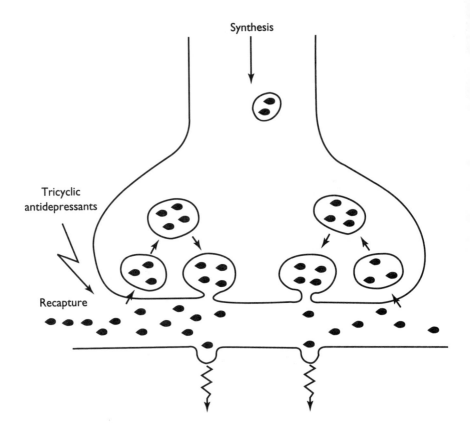

Figure 2.13   Mono-amine neurotransmission at a neuronal synapse (norepinephrine or serotonin/5HT). Tricyclics potentiate two descending inhibitory pathways from the brain (one noradrenergic, the other serotonergic) by blocking presynaptic re-uptake. They also potentiate opioid analgesia by a serotonergic mechanism in the brain stem.

Anticonvulsant

e.g. sodium valproate 200–1000 mg nocte or carbamazepine

Carbamazepine is more difficult to use than sodium valproate. Although the plasma halflife of a single dose is about 36 h, this reduces to 16–24 h as a result of hepatic enzyme induction by carbamazepine itself and by concurrently administered anticonvulsants. Plasma concentrations increase significantly after each dose even when a steady-state is attained – sufficient to cause or exacerbate adverse effects.[35] Diplopia, drowsiness and headache are the most common adverse effects; nystagmus and ataxia may also occur.[36] It is better to give carbamazepine in a lower dose more frequently than a higher dose less often, e.g. 50–100 mg q.d.s. initially, rather than 100–200 mg b.d. M/r preparations are best taken b.d. Increments should generally be restricted to 200 mg/week.

- dextropropoxyphene (in co-proxamol) enhances the action of carbamazepine
- some SSRIs increase plasma carbamazepine and plasma valproic acid concentrations; paroxetine does not
- the metabolism of tricyclic antidepressants is accelerated by carbamazepine but, even so, tricyclics antagonize the anticonvulsant action of carbamazepine by lowering the convulsive threshold
- the metabolism of tricyclic antidepressants is inhibited by sodium valproate.

Anti-arrhythmic

e.g. flecainide 50–150 mg b.d. or mexiletine 50–300 mg t.d.s.

The main disadvantage is the negative inotropic effect on the heart. *Should not be given to patients with evidence of cardiac failure.* Toxicity includes confusion, paraesthesiae, multifocal myoclonus, fitting and coma. Use smaller doses in renal failure. Risk of pro-arrhythmic effect if used with a tricyclic.

Expectations

About 90% of patients respond well to step 1–3 drugs (Figure 2.10); the rest require spinal analgesia or other measures to obtain adequate relief.

The response is not an 'all or none' phenomenon. The crucial first step in many cases is to help the patient obtain a good night's sleep with step 1 or step 2 drugs. The second is to reduce pain intensity and allodynia to a bearable level during the day. Initially, benefit may be for only part of each day. Adverse effects tend to be the limiting therapeutic factor.

The patient should be warned that results often take a week or more to become apparent, although improvement in sleep should occur immediately.

Sympathetically maintained pain

Occasionally a cancer patient presents with an opioid-resistant pain which is dependent on the integrity of the sympathetic nerves. In other words, a regional sympathetic nerve block relieves the pain. The block possibly works by interrupting abnormal activity between (efferent) sympathetic nerve terminals and (afferent) somatic nerve receptors.

Sympathetically maintained pain is more likely when the malignant process involves the sympathetic chain. This is seen mostly with

- invasion of a nerve plexus
- malignant lymph glands in the neck
- mesothelioma
- cancer of the cervix uteri.

The hand and forearm is the most frequently affected area.

There are two distinct pain components

- a superficial burning pain with allodynia
- a deep aching posturally dependent pain which resolves with limb or head elevation.

The co-existence of circulatory, sweating and trophic changes together with allodynia are diagnostic of sympathetically maintained pain.

Evaluation

The essential features are

- pain (often burning)
- sensory disorder (nondermatomal, often extensive and circumferential)
- relief following a sympathetic block.

It is necessary to differentiate between the burning pain of de-afferentation and the burning pain of a sympathetically maintained pain. This can be difficult as features are not constant and the two may co-exist (Table 2.14). Note that

- there may be radiographic evidence of osteoporosis and of hot spots on isotope bone scans which may be mistaken for osteolytic metastases

Table 2.14   Superficial burning pain

	Somatic de-afferentation	Sympathetically maintained
Pattern	Dermatomal (if peripheral)	Nondermatomal
Characteristic	Not cold sensitive	Cold sensitive
Concomitants		
stabbing pain	Common	Uncommon
allodynia and hyperpathia[a]	Typical	Typical
deep pressure	May relieve	Exacerbates
pinprick	Variable response	Diminished response
muscle atrophy	+	+/–
muscle fatigue	Not obvious	Marked
trophic changes	Late	Early[b]
limb temperature	Cool if limb not used	Usually cold but sometimes hot with vasodilation
Tricyclic drug	Beneficial	Ineffective
Sympathetic block	No relief	Relief

a   *see* p.57

b   trophic changes may affect skin, subcutaneous tissues and/or nails; may be atrophic (e.g. shiny taut skin, hair loss) or hypertrophic (e.g. hyperkeratosis).

- the distribution of sympathetically maintained pain does not correspond with the dermatomal pattern of the peripheral nerves. Instead it reflects the pattern of sympathetic vascular innervation (Figure 2.14).

Treatment

If sympathetically maintained pain is suspected, arrangements should be made for the patient to have a diagnostic sympathetic block with local anaesthetic. This serves not only to confirm the diagnosis but may also give relief which outlasts the duration of action of the local anaesthetic. A lumbar chemical sympathectomy is of benefit in most patients with lower limb pain.

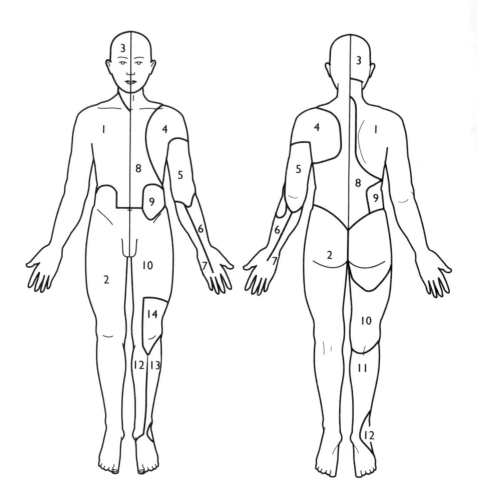

Figure 2.14   Arterial supply of the skin.[37]
1 subclavian artery = cervicothoracic trunk outflow = upper quadrant of the body;
2 iliac arteries = lumbar sympathetic outflow = lower quadrant of the body;
3 common carotid artery; 4 axillary artery; 5 brachial artery; 6 radial artery;
7 ulnar artery; 8 thoracic aorta; 9 abdominal aorta; 10 femoral artery;
11 popliteal artery; 12 posterior tibial artery; 13 anterior tibial artery.

Common mistakes in cancer pain management

- failure to distinguish between pains caused by cancer and pain related to other causes

- failure to evaluate each pain individually and to plan separate treatments if necessary

- failure to use nondrug treatments, particularly for muscle spasm pain
- lack of awareness that some pains are not relieved by opioid analgesics and that others require combined treatment with morphine and a second drug
- *laissez-faire* approach to drug time-table and education of patient and family
- changing to an alternative analgesic before optimizing the dose and timing of the previous analgesic
- combining analgesics inappropriately, e.g. two weak opioids or a strong opioid and a weak opioid
- belief that pentazocine is more effective than codeine and related drugs
- failure to appreciate that a mixed agonist-antagonist such as pentazocine should not be used together with codeine and morphine
- reluctance to prescribe morphine
- changing from an alternative strong opioid (e.g. buprenorphine, oxycodone) to a smaller equivalent dose of morphine
- reducing the interval between administrations instead of increasing the dose
- using injections when oral medication is possible
- failure to monitor and manage adverse effects, particularly constipation
- lack of attention to psychosocial issues
- failure to listen to the patient.

Useful definitions

Pharmacological terms

Receptor affinity ('potency')	A term used to describe the power of attraction between the drug and the drug receptor. Affinity determines the dose of drug required to produce a certain level of biological effect.
Intrinsic activity ('efficacy')	The degree to which the drug is able to stimulate a receptor and thereby produce a biological effect. Intrinsic activity is a basic property of all drugs which act through receptors.
Full agonist	A drug which when bound to the receptor stimulates the receptor to the maximum level, e.g. morphine. By definition the intrinsic activity of a full agonist is unity.
Pure antagonist	A drug which when bound to the receptor fails completely to produce any stimulation of that receptor, e.g. naloxone. By definition the intrinsic activity of a pure antagonist is zero.
Partial agonist	A drug which when bound to the receptor stimulates the receptor to a level below the maximum level, e.g. buprenorphine (partial mu agonist). By definition the intrinsic activity of a partial agonist lies between zero and unity.
Mixed agonist-antagonist	A drug which acts simultaneously on different types of receptor, with the potential for agonist action on one or more types and antagonist action on one or more types, e.g. pentazocine (partial mu agonist + kappa agonist + weak delta antagonist).
Ligand	A substance which binds to a receptor. The use of this term circumvents the need to say whether the substance is an agonist or an antagonist.

Pain terms[38]

Allodynia	Pain caused by a stimulus which does not normally provoke pain.
Anaesthesia dolorosa	Pain in an area which is numb.
Analgesia	Absence of pain in response to stimulation which would normally be painful.
Causalgia	A syndrome of sustained burning pain, allodynia and hyperpathia after a traumatic nerve lesion, often combined with vasomotor and sudomotor dysfunction and later trophic changes.
Central pain	Pain associated with a lesion of the CNS.
Dysaesthesia	An unpleasant abnormal sensation, whether spontaneous or evoked.
Hyperaesthesia	Increased sensitivity to stimulation.
Hyperalgesia	An increased response to a stimulus which is normally painful.
Hyperpathia	A painful syndrome characterized by increased reaction to a stimulus, especially a repetitive stimulus, *as well as an increased threshold*. (This latter feature results in a delayed onset. It tends to be poorly localized and outlasts the stimulus.)
Neuralgia	Pain in the distribution of a nerve.
Neuropathy	A disturbance of function or pathological change in a nerve.
Nociceptor	A receptor preferentially sensitive to a noxious stimulus or to a stimulus which would become noxious if prolonged.
Noxious stimulus	A noxious stimulus is one which is damaging to normal tissues.
Pain	An unpleasant sensory and emotional experience associated with actual or potential tissue damage or described in terms of such damage.
Pain threshold	The least experience of pain which a subject can recognize.
Pain tolerance level	The greatest level of pain which a subject is prepared to tolerate.

References

1   Travell J and Rinzler SH (1952) The myofascial genesis of pain. *Postgraduate Medicine (Minneapolis).* **11 May**: 425–434.

2   Grond S *et al.* (1996) Assessment of cancer pain: a prospective evaluation in 2266 cancer patients referred to a pain service. *Pain.* **64**: 107–114.

3   Hoskin PJ (1988) Scientific and clinical aspects of radiotherapy in the relief of bone pain. In: GW Hanks (ed) *Cancer Surveys. Vol 7, no. 1.* Oxford University Press, Oxford. pp 69–86.

4   World Health Organization (1986) *Cancer pain relief.* WHO, Geneva.

5   Eriksson L-O *et al.* (1990) Effects of sulindac and naproxen on prostaglandin excretion in patients with impaired renal function and rheumatoid arthritis. *American Journal of Medicine.* **89**: 313–321.

6   Guth B *et al.* (1996) Therapeutic doses of meloxicam do not inhibit platelet aggregation in man. *Rheumatology in Europe.* **25** (Suppl 1): Abs 443.

7   Cullen L *et al.* (1997) Selective suppression of cyclo-oxygenase-2 during chronic administration of nimesulide in man. *Presented at 4th International Congress on essential fatty acids and eicosanoids.* Edinburgh.

8   MacDonald TM (1994) Selected side-effects: 14. Non-steroidal anti-inflammatory drugs and renal damage. *Prescribers' Journal.* **34**: 77–80.

9   Sindrup SH *et al.* (1992) The effect of quinidine on the analgesic effect of codeine. *European Journal of Clinical Pharmacology.* **42**: 587–592.

10 Regnard C (1987) Opioids, sleep and the time of death. *Palliative Medicine.* **1**: 107–110.

11 Hanks G *et al.* (1996) Morphine in cancer pain: modes of administration. *British Medical Journal.* **312**: 823–826.

12 Bruera E *et al.* (1996) Opioid rotation in patients with cancer pain. *Cancer.* **78**: 852–857.

13 Gorman AL *et al.* (1997) The d- and l-isomers of methadone bind to the non-competitive site on the N-methyl-D-aspartate (NMDA) receptor in rat forebrain and spinal cord. *Neuroscience Letters.* **223**: 5–8.

14 Glare PA and Walsh TD (1993) Dose-ranging study of oxycodone for chronic pain in advanced cancer. *Journal of Clinical Oncology.* **11**: 973–978.

15 Poyhia R *et al.* (1993) Oxycodone: an alternative to morphine for cancer pain. A review. *Journal of Pain and Symptom Management.* **8**: 63–67.

16 Kaiko R *et al.* (1996a) Clinical pharmacokinetics of controlled-release oxycodone in renal impairment. *Clinical Pharmacology and Therapeutics.* **59**: 130.

17 Heiskanen T *et al.* (1996) Double-blind, randomised, repeated dose, crossover comparison of controlled-release oxycodone and controlled-release morphine in cancer pain. 1: pharmacodynamic profile. *Abstracts of 8th World Congress on Pain.* IASP Press, Seattle. pp 17–18.

18 Kaiko R *et al.* (1996b) Analgesic onset and potency of oral controlled-release (CR) oxycodone and controlled-release morphine. *Clinical Pharmacology and Therapeutics.* **59**: 130.

19 McDonald CJ and Miller AJ (1997) A comparative potency study of a controlled release tablet formulation of hydromorphone with controlled release morphine

in patients with cancer pain. *Presented at 5th Congress of the European Association for Palliative Care.*

20   TTS-fentanyl Multicentre Study Group (1994) Transdermal fentanyl in cancer pain. *Journal of Drug Development.* **6**: 93–97.

21   Gourlay GK *et al.* (1989) The transdermal administration of fentanyl in the treatment of post-operative pain: pharmacokinetics and pharmacodynamic effects. *Pain.* **37**: 193–202.

22   Portenoy RK *et al.* (1993) Transdermal fentanyl for cancer pain. *Anesthesiology.* **78**: 36–43.

23   Hammack JE and Loprinzi CL (1994) Use of orally administered opioids for cancer-related pain. *Mayo Clinic Proceedings.* **69**: 384–390.

24   Donner B *et al.* (1996) Direct conversion from oral morphine to transdermal fentanyl: a multicenter study in patients with cancer pain. *Pain.* **64**: 527–534.

25   Ahmedzai S and Brooks D (1997) Transdermal fentanyl versus sustained-release oral morphine in cancer pain: preference, efficacy, and quality of life. *Journal of Pain and Symptom Management.* **13**: 254–261.

26   Herz A and Teschmacher H-J (1971) Activities and sites of antinociceptive action of morphine-like analgesics and kinetics of distribution following intravenous, intracerebral and intraventricular application. *Advances in Drug Research.* **6**: 79–119.

27   Korbon GA *et al.* (1985) Intramuscular naloxone reverses the side effects of epidural morphine while preserving analgesia. *Regional Anesthesia.* **10**: 16–20.

28   Max MB and Payne R (Co-chairs). *Principles of analgesic use in the treatment of acute pain and cancer pain.* American Pain Society, 1992, p.41.

29   McQuay HJ *et al.* (1995) Anti-convulsant drugs for management of pain: a systematic review. *British Medical Journal.* **311**: 1047–1052.

30   McQuay HJ *et al.* (1996) A systematic review of antidepressants in neuropathic pain. *Pain.* **68**: 217–227.

31   Luczak J *et al.* (1995) A role of ketamine, an NMDA receptor antagonist, in the management of pain. *Progress in Palliative Care.* **3**: 127–134.

32   Fallon MT and Welsh J (1996) The role of ketamine in pain control. *European Journal of Palliative Care.* **3**: 143–146.

33   Clark JL and Kalan GE (1995) Effective treatment of severe cancer pain in the head using low-dose ketamine in an opioid-tolerant patient. *Journal of Pain and Symptom Management.* **10**: 310–314.

34   Broadley KE *et al.* (1996) Ketamine injection used orally. *Palliative Medicine.* **10**: 247–250.

35   Tomson T (1984) Interdosage fluctuations in plasma carbamazepine concentration determine intermittent side effects. *Archives of Neurology.* **41**: 830-834.

36   Hoppener RJ *et al.* (1980) Correlation between daily fluctuations of carbamazepine serum levels and intermittent side effects. *Epilepsia.* **21**: 341–350.

37   Gerbershagen HU (1979) Blocks with local anesthetics in the treatment of cancer pain. In: JJ Bonica and V Ventafridda (eds) *Advances in Pain Research and Therapy. Vol 2.* Raven Press, New York. pp 313–323.

38   International Association for the Study of Pain Task Force on Taxonomy (1994) *Classification of chronic pain.* (2nd edn) IASP Press, Seattle.

3   Oral morphine in advanced cancer

Oral morphine

1   What are the indications for morphine in advanced cancer?

Main

- pain
- dyspnoea (*see* p.90).

Subsidiary

- cough
- diarrhoea.

Note: Sedation is *not* an indication for morphine.

2   Why use morphine? What about other strong opioids?

Morphine is a versatile drug. By mouth, it has a plasma halflife of 2–2.5 h and, apart from patients with renal failure, there is no danger of drug cumulation. By mouth, no other strong opioid shows a clear advantage over morphine. Transdermal fentanyl, however, has advantages both in terms of ease of administration and less constipation.

Oxycodone and hydromorphone may be regarded as morphine 'look-alikes', although in some patients they have fewer adverse effects. Levorphanol and phenazocine have longer plasma halflives and generally need to be given only q6h–q8h; methadone only q8h–q12h. Phenazocine is available only as 5 mg tablets. This is equivalent to 20–25 mg of oral morphine and many patients do not need as much as this.

3   What is the best way of giving morphine by mouth?

In practice, the choice is between a solution or tablet of morphine sulphate/ hydrochloride and m/r tablets or suspension. Morphine solution and ordinary tablets are administered q4h; m/r tablets q12h or o.d. and m/r suspension q12h. Some pharmacies produce their own morphine solutions.

At some centres m/r tablets are considered the formulation of choice, while at others morphine solution or ordinary tablets are preferred. The convenience of a q12h regimen compared with q4h makes the m/r morphine an attractive option, particularly for those at home.

Initial dose titration with morphine solution or ordinary tablets is advisable in patients with a history of poor pain management. At some centres, m/r tablets q12h are used from the start.

Response to morphine

4   In relation to pain, when should morphine be used?

From a therapeutic point of view, pain in cancer can be divided into three categories

• morphine-responsive, i.e. pain relieved by morphine

• morphine-semiresponsive, i.e. pain relieved by the concurrent use of morphine *and* an adjuvant drug (co-analgesic)

• morphine-resistant, i.e. pain that is not relieved by morphine.

For morphine-responsive pains, morphine should be prescribed when a weak opioid (i.e. codeine, dextropropoxyphene or dihydrocodeine) fails to relieve the pain.

Although functional gastro-intestinal pains are morphine-responsive, they should be treated more specifically

• gastric distension:
   dietary advice
   antiflatulent
   prokinetic drug

• irritable bowel syndrome:
   antispasmodic
   bulk-forming agent

- constipation:
    laxative
    enema.

These are morphine-responsive pains for which morphine should not be used.

5 Which pains are only semiresponsive to morphine?

The following pains are generally only *semiresponsive* to morphine

- bone and soft tissue metastasis
- raised intracranial pressure
- nerve compression and nerve injury.

A partial response calls for adjuvant medication and consideration of non-drug treatments

- bone and soft tissue pain:
    NSAID
    radiotherapy (treatment of choice for bone pain)
- raised intracranial pressure and nerve compression:
    corticosteroid
- nerve injury:
    antidepressant
    anticonvulsant (*see* p.46).

Pain caused by lumbosacral plexopathy is often best treated with epidural morphine and bupivacaine, or with SC ketamine and oral morphine. The pain from superficial bedsores is also only semiresponsive to morphine. Here, care in movement plays an important role in management.

6 What do you mean by morphine-resistant pains?

The following pains should be regarded as *morphine-resistant* and require alternative specific treatments

- headache:
    tension
    migraine
- cramp (muscle spasm).

Movement-related pain often does not respond well to oral morphine. So much morphine is required for relief during activity that the patient becomes unacceptably drowsy at rest. The dose of morphine is therefore titrated against rest pain rather than movement-related pain. (Some centres use subcutaneous patient-controlled analgesia (PCA) pumps in this situation to good effect.)

7   Are there any other important morphine-resistant pains?

There are several other circumstances in which pain *appears* to be morphine-resistant.

These include

- underdosing:
    too small
    too infrequent
    given as needed
- poor alimentary absorption (rare)
- ignoring psychological, social and spiritual factors.

8   Can psychological factors really inhibit the action of morphine?

Morphine (or any other opioid) should be given only within the context of comprehensive biopsychosocial care. If psychological factors are ignored, pain may well prove intractable.

A 55 year old man with recently diagnosed cancer of the oesophagus was still in pain despite receiving m/r morphine tablets *6000 mg* (100 mg × 60) b.d. Following inpatient admission to a palliative care unit, he became painfree on *30 mg* b.d. and diazepam 10 mg nocte. He returned home, converted the spare bedroom into a workshop, and was able to spend many happy hours there. The key to success was *physical and psychological evaluation, explanation and setting positive rehabilitation goals.*

The first step is to break the vicious circle of pain, sleeplessness, exhaustion, increasing pain and increasing distress. Achieving a good night's sleep initially may require a night sedative or anxiolytic as well as morphine.

An antidepressant should be prescribed if the patient is clinically depressed. It may not be easy to distinguish between exhaustion stemming from long continued pain and insomnia and depression. With pains expected to respond to morphine, lack of success is one pointer to depression (*see* p.100).

9 Can I ever be confident that the use of morphine will result in complete relief?

Yes – if the pain is morphine-responsive. Partial relief obtained with a weak opioid or when morphine is first prescribed often indicates whether the pain is morphine-responsive.

Doctor	'When you take your tablets (weak opioid), how soon do you get relief?'
Patient	'After 20–30 minutes.'
Doctor	'How long does the relief last?'
Patient	'About 1½–2 hours.'
Doctor	'How much of the pain is relieved by the tablets? 25%, 50%, 75%?'
Patient	'I would say about 50%; they make it bearable.'
Doctor	'That's good, because it tells me that you have a pain which responds to this type of painkiller. What we need to do now is to use something stronger to get rid of at least 95% of your pain.'

In this situation, the doctor can be confident that the use of morphine will achieve greater, possibly complete, relief.

Starting treatment with morphine

10 What are the basic principles governing the use of morphine in advanced cancer?

- an adjuvant drug or a nondrug treatment will be necessary if the pain is only semiresponsive to morphine

- use within the context of comprehensive biopsychosocial care
- administer by the mouth
- administer by the clock
- adjust the dose to individual need
- anticipate and treat vomiting and constipation
- monitor response.

11   Is it better to start treatment with morphine solution/ordinary tablets or with m/r tablets?

It is often easier to begin with morphine solution or ordinary tablets q4h and convert to m/r tablets when the dose has stabilized. This is not an absolute rule, however, and some centres titrate with m/r morphine backed up with *rescue doses* of morphine solution or ordinary tablets (*see* Question 17).

12   How do I decide on the initial dose of oral morphine?

If weak opioids have not been used or small doses only (e.g. codeine 30 mg q4h), 5–6 mg q4h (or m/r morphine 15 mg q12h) may be adequate. If the patient has been taking the equivalent of codeine 60 mg q4h, 10 mg q4h (or m/r morphine 30 mg q12h) is the correct starting dose.

If the weak opioid has been taken only t.d.s. or q.d.s. as needed and has given good, though intermittent, relief, the first step may be not to prescribe morphine but to take the weak opioid regularly q4h. If the patient is painfree the next day, the regular use of the weak opioid q4h should be continued; *morphine is not indicated.* If the patient is only 75–90% comfortable, treatment with morphine should be started.

13   What about the patient who is taking an alternative strong opioid?

All strong opioids can be regarded as alternatives to morphine and substitute effectively for morphine in the appropriate dose. The important exceptions to this rule are

- buprenorphine (a partial mu agonist)
- pethidine/meperidine.

Both buprenorphine and pethidine have an analgesic ceiling dose above which no further benefit is obtained. The ceiling for SL buprenorphine is probably between 3–5 mg/24 h. This is equivalent to a total daily dose of 180–300 mg of oral morphine.

With pethidine the ceiling is related to adverse effects (tremor, twitching, fits, agitation) caused by norpethidine, a toxic metabolite. Total daily doses should be limited to 600 mg, and ideally, it should not be used for more than 48 h. Toxic manifestations occur with lower doses in patients with poor renal function.

With other strong opioids, if the patient has previously had good relief but is now 'getting used to the tablets', it may just be necessary to increase the dose in order to re-establish good relief.

A decision to change to morphine may be made because

- of unacceptable drowsiness, or

- it has been necessary to take the alternative drug q2h–q3h because it is short acting, e.g. pethidine and dextromoramide.

14 Is morphine 10 mg q4h the right starting dose for a patient previously receiving an alternative strong opioid?

No! If morphine 10 mg q4h (or m/r morphine 30 mg b.d.) is prescribed in these circumstances, the patient will soon be in severe pain. This is unnecessary and damages the morale of both patient and family. It may also lead to the false conclusion that 'morphine is no good for Mr Smith's pain: it doesn't work for him.'

This is particularly relevant in the USA, where oxycodone is often used in combination with a nonopioid analgesic – Percodan, Percocet and Tylox. These contain 5 mg of oxycodone together with either aspirin or paracetamol. It is not always appreciated that by mouth oxycodone 5 mg is equivalent to morphine 6–7 mg.

15 What is the right starting dose for patients changing from an alternative strong opioid?

The dose of morphine to be prescribed is calculated as follows

- add up the total 24 h dose of the alternative strong opioid

- multiply this by the potency of the strong opioid in question (Table 3.1). This is the *total daily dose of morphine* which will give comparable relief

Table 3.1   Approximate oral analgesic equivalence to morphine[a]

Analgesic	Potency ratio with morphine	Duration of action (h)[b]
Codeine } Dihydrocodeine	1/10	3–5
Pethidine (meperidine USA)	1/8	2–3
Tramadol	1/5[c]	5–6
Dipipanone (in Diconal UK)	1/2	3–5
Papaveretum	2/3[d]	3–5
Oxycodone	1.5–2[c]	5–6
Dextromoramide	[2][e]	2–3
Levorphanol	5	6–8
Phenazocine	5	6–8
Methadone	5–10[f]	8–12
Hydromorphone	7.5	3–5
Buprenorphine (sublingual)	60	6–8
Fentanyl (transdermal)	150	72

a   multiply dose of opioid by its potency ratio to determine the equivalent dose of morphine sulphate

b   dependent in part on severity of pain and on dose; often longer lasting in very elderly and those with renal dysfunction

c   tramadol and oxycodone are both relatively more potent by mouth because of high bio-availability; parenteral potency ratios with morphine are 1/10 and 3/4 respectively

d   papaveretum (strong opium) is standardized to contain 50% morphine base; potency expressed in relation to morphine sulphate

e   dextromoramide: a single 5 mg dose is equivalent to morphine 15 mg in terms of peak effect but is shorter acting; overall potency ratio adjusted accordingly

f   methadone: a single 5 mg dose is equivalent to morphine 7.5 mg. Has a plasma halflife of 8–80 h which leads to cumulation in many patients when given repeatedly; overall potency ratio adjusted accordingly. Methadone also has a broader spectrum of receptor site affinities and may relieve pain which is responding poorly to very high doses of morphine (e.g. 1 g or more in 24 h) with relatively much smaller doses.

- if the patient has been in pain despite the use of the alternative strong opioid, the total daily dose of morphine should be increased by 30–50%

- if using ordinary morphine tablets or solution, divide the calculated total daily dose by 6 and round up to the nearest convenient 5 mg or 10 mg. This is the correct q4h starting dose of morphine – which could be 60 mg or even more

- if using m/r tablets, divide by 2 and round up to the nearest convenient b.d. dose – which could be as much as 200 mg.

16   Overwhelming pain

Some patients present a picture of, 'It's all pain, doctor.' They are often highly anxious, demoralized, and exhausted from pain-related insomnia. In this situation there is no way of estimating what a patient will need to achieve relief.

Initially an anxiolytic (e.g. diazepam) and morphine should be prescribed concurrently. The nurses should be instructed to repeat the initial combined medication after 1 h if the patient is not much more comfortable. Review by the doctor after 2 h and 4 h is not excessive. Subsequent doses of both drugs depend on the initial response.

Overwhelming pain is generally the result of weeks or months of unrelieved severe pain. *It should be regarded as a medical emergency.* Best results are obtained if *one doctor* (or at most two) accepts responsibility for frequent review and prescribing. Spinal cord compression may cause widespread pain in the lower half of the body and must be distinguished from the syndrome of overwhelming pain.

17   How soon should a patient be re-evaluated after starting oral morphine?

Ideally after 2 h and again after 4 h! This is rarely possible if the patient is at home. Monitoring progress must be seen as the shared responsibility of the patient, family, nurses and doctor. Provided that each one knows his or her part, it is unlikely that anything will go seriously wrong.

The patient and family should be advised that the starting dose may not completely relieve the pain. Various strategies can be adopted to cope with this. The most straightforward is to advise the patient, if necessary, to use an extra *rescue dose* between the regular doses:

'If the morphine solution/tablet does not give more than 75% relief, take a *rescue dose* after 2 h. If you do this, you must still take the next regular dose on time.' (Here the rescue dose will be the *same* as the regular q4h dose.) *or*

'If the effect of the m/r tablets wears off in less than 12 h, take a *rescue dose* of morphine solution or ordinary tablets.' (Here the rescue dose will be approximately *one third* of the q12h dose.)

The aim is to increase the regular dose progressively until the patient's pain is relieved (dose titration). The patient should therefore be advised to increase the dose by 30–50% on the second day if the pain is not 90% relieved (even if he feels moderately drowsy), and again 2–3 days later.

As the regular dose increases, the need for rescue doses decreases. Rescue doses, however, are a continuing part of pain management. After every dose adjustment the patient should be told what is the right rescue dose for him.

18   What other general advice should a patient be given?

It is important to tell the patient:

'If you are unhappy about the new medication, contact me at ... (name and telephone number of doctor or nurse)' *or*

'I (or nurse) will be in touch later today/tomorrow to review progress' *or*

'Would you phone me tomorrow to let me know how things are going?'

When an unknown team member is to be on duty; give the patient the name of the person and a few words of introduction and re-assurance:

'Dr X/Nurse Y is on call tonight. We work closely together, and I will tell him/her about you before I go off duty.'

It should be exceptional for a patient not to be visited on the second day of treatment by either a doctor or nurse familiar with oral morphine therapy. The dose of morphine may need to be adjusted, particularly during the first few days.

The patient and family often have many questions they wish to ask about the use of morphine, e.g. 'Will I become addicted?' Professional time must be made for discussion.

Professional support is necessary to encourage the patient and family during the period of initial adverse effects. Also, only the trained professional can recognize when the dose of morphine should be reduced temporarily or when morphine intolerance cannot be circumvented (*see* Question 36).

It is irresponsible to prescribe morphine and not make arrangements for close supervision by somebody familiar with its use.

19   How soon should the patient become painfree?

Total immediate success is a bonus. It is best, therefore, to agree on a series of sequential goals

- a good night's sleep free of pain – normally achieved in 2–3 days
- comfort at rest (sitting or lying) during the day – normally achieved in 3–5 days
- comfort when active – normally achieved in 3–7 days. In patients with multiple vertebral or pelvic metastases, this third level of relief may not be possible
- for patients with persisting movement-related pain, suggest ways in which the patient might modify his way of life so as to reduce activities which cause or exacerbate pain.

In patients with more than one pain, each pain should be re-evaluated. Some respond more readily than others. Re-evaluation remains a continuing necessity. Old pains may get worse and new ones may develop.

If the patient is very anxious or depressed, it may take 3–4 weeks to achieve a satisfactory result.

20   What should be done if the chosen dose of morphine does not completely relieve the patient's pain?

If there is little relief after one or two increments, it is possible that the patient has a morphine-resistant pain. In this circumstance, an alternative strategy is necessary.

Alternatively, a poor response may indicate that the pain has a higher than average psychological component. This will demand more time, more psycho-therapeutic support and possibly the prescription of an anxiolytic or an antidepressant.

21   By how much should the dose of morphine be increased?

A 50% increase is generally appropriate; certainly no less than 33%. Each adjustment takes time, and time and confidence are lost if an adjustment yields little benefit. It is important to be equally decisive when increasing the dose of m/r tablets.

Coping with adverse effects

22   What are the common adverse effects of morphine?

Initial

- vomiting
- drowsiness
- unsteadiness
- confusion (delirium).

Continuing

- constipation.

Occasional

- dry mouth
- sweating
- myoclonus.

Note: Addiction and respiratory depression are *not* listed (*see* Question 34 and Question 35).

23   Is the use of morphine limited by adverse effects?

- generally no
- occasionally yes.

Adverse effects are minimized by close supervision and by the use of an appropriate anti-emetic and a laxative.

24   Is an anti-emetic always necessary?

If the patient vomits after taking morphine, the morphine will not be absorbed, the patient remains in pain, and confidence in the new medicine is lost. To avoid this, some doctors use an anti-emetic routinely when morphine is prescribed.

Although this is good advice for the inexperienced prescriber, once a doctor and the team feel confident in the use of oral morphine, a more selective approach is possible.

The following patients should be prescribed an anti-emetic prophylactically

- those who are already experiencing nausea and vomiting from another cause

- those who are experiencing nausea and vomiting with codeine or other weak opioid

- those who vomited when given a strong opioid in the past.

The following patients need not be prescribed an anti-emetic prophylactically

- those with no nausea and vomiting

- those taking a weak or alternative strong analgesic regularly without nausea or vomiting.

One third of all patients prescribed morphine never need an anti-emetic.

25   Which anti-emetic is best?

This depends on whether morphine is the main or only cause of the vomiting (*see* p.195). If caused by morphine, haloperidol 1–1.5 mg PO stat and nocte is generally satisfactory. Occasionally a twice daily regimen may be better, e.g. 0.5–1.5 mg PO b.d.

Fluphenazine 0.5–2 mg PO b.d. is equally effective but is little used in the UK because, unlike haloperidol, there is no parenteral formulation available.

26   Are there circumstances in which haloperidol or fluphenazine fail to relieve morphine-induced vomiting?

Yes. Although stimulation of the chemoreceptor trigger zone in the brain stem is the commonest cause of morphine-induced vomiting, morphine can precipitate vomiting by other mechanisms

- delayed gastric emptying

- secondary to constipation

- vestibular disturbance.

Vomiting secondary to delayed gastric emptying is a problem in <10% of patients prescribed oral morphine. It is reminiscent of pyloric stenosis. The use of a prokinetic anti-emetic (i.e. metoclopramide or domperidone 10 mg q4h) generally permits the continued use of morphine. If necessary the dose of metoclopramide or domperidone should be increased to 20 mg q4h for 1 week. Alternatively, cisapride 20 mg b.d. can be prescribed instead.

27   Can the anti-emetic be stopped?

Vomiting with morphine is mainly an initial effect. If an anti-emetic was prescribed prophylactically, and not to relieve pre-existing nausea and vomiting, it is good practice to stop it after the patient has been on a steady dose of morphine for 1 week. Remember that one third of patients receiving morphine never need an anti-emetic. If necessary, the anti-emetic can be restarted.

28   Do patients become drowsy on morphine?

Like nausea and vomiting, drowsiness tends to be troublesome during the first few days, and subsequently if the dose is increased. Patients should be warned about initial drowsiness and encouraged to persevere in the knowledge that it will lessen after a few more days. Occasionally, in the elderly and frail patient, it is necessary to reduce the dose of morphine and then increase it again more slowly, every 2–3 days, until adequate relief is obtained.

29   Do some patients go on feeling very drowsy and drugged?

Occasionally, yes (Table 3.2). It is important to distinguish between persistent drowsiness and inactivity or boredom drowsiness. Most patients receiving morphine catnap with ease. This means that they will drop off to sleep if sitting quietly and alone. As many of these patients have little stamina, they need more rest and sleep than when healthy.

Provided that they are easily roused and can converse readily when joined by family or friends, continuing inactivity drowsiness should be seen as a bonus. Indeed many patients find that it helps to pass what otherwise might be a long and exhausting day.

If stamina is not limited, the patient can live a normal active life because any continuing drowsiness is related to inactivity.

Table 3.2   Checklist for excessive drowsiness in patients receiving oral morphine

---

General factors

Is the patient still recuperating from prolonged fatigue?

Is the patient more ill than I thought?

renal failure	hepatic failure
hypercalcaemia	cerebral metastases
hyponatraemia	septicaemia
hyperglycaemia	cardiac failure

Drug factors

Is the patient completely painfree?
If yes, reduce the dose and review both drowsiness and pain relief

Is the patient on a psychotropic drug, notably a benzodiazepine (e.g. diazepam) or a phenothiazine (e.g. chlorpromazine)? Is it necessary?

If no, cut it out
If yes, can the dose be reduced?

If the patient is taking a phenothiazine anti-emetic, can it be changed to haloperidol or metoclopramide?

Patients with renal failure are particularly likely to become drowsy because of cumulation of an active metabolite, morphine-6-glucuronide. This necessitates a reduction in dose of morphine.

Moderate hepatic insufficiency does *not* affect the metabolism of morphine; severe hepatic failure does, and may necessitate a reduction in dose.

If drowsiness continues to be a problem, an alternative strong opioid should be considered (*see* p.34).

30   Do patients become confused?

Yes, a few. Particularly the elderly who are more sensitive to the effects of morphine. It will be necessary to titrate the dose of morphine more slowly in these patients, possibly starting on a lower dose or prescribing q6h–q8h initially. Those over 70 years old should be warned that they may become muddled at times during the first few days, but to persevere.

Confusion (delirium) may be caused by the concurrent use of morphine and psychotropic drugs and/or anticholinergic drugs. If confusional symptoms persist, a reduction in concurrent medication should be considered (Table 3.2).

31 Is postural hypotension a problem?

No. Advise those over 70 years old that they may experience dizziness or feel unsteady for a few days, but to persevere.

32 Constipation

This is the most troublesome adverse effect of treatment with morphine. Almost all patients become constipated unless they have an ileostomy or steatorrhoea. If not corrected, a patient may stop his medication and suffer severe pain rather than continue to be severely constipated.

An appropriate laxative should be prescribed when morphine is started (Box 3.A). *Correcting constipation may be more difficult than relieving pain.*

In cases of severe continuing constipation, switching to transdermal fentanyl will be beneficial (*see* p.39).

33 Sweating

Some patients complain of sweating. This can be profuse and tends to be more troublesome at night. It occurs more in patients with liver metastases. Sleeping lightly clad in a cool room may be all that one can suggest to the patient. Most patients put up with the sweating as an acceptable price to pay for freedom from pain, particularly when they understand that it has no sinister meaning.

Sweating may also be troublesome in patients with a fever caused by the cancer. In this case, benefit may be obtained from the concurrent prescription of a NSAID.

34 What about addiction?

Psychological dependence (addiction) does not occur in patients prescribed morphine for cancer pain, provided it is used within the context of total patient care.

Occasionally, a patient is admitted who appears to be addicted, demanding an injection q2h–q3h. Typically such a patient has a long history of poor pain management, and for several weeks will have been receiving fairly regular (q4h as needed) but inadequate injections of one or more opioid analgesics.

Box 3.A Management of opioid-induced constipation

Ask about the patient's normal bowel habit and use of laxatives; record date of last bowel action.

Do a rectal examination if faecal impaction is suspected or if the patient reports diarrhoea or faecal incontinence (to exclude impaction with overflow).

For inpatients, record bowel actions each day in a Bowel Book.

Encourage fluids generally, and fruit juice, fruit and bran specifically.

When an opioid is first prescribed, prescribe co-danthrusate[a] I capsule nocte prophylactically.

If already constipated, prescribe co-danthrusate 2 capsules nocte.

Adjust the dose every few days according to results, up to 3 capsules t.d.s.

If the patient prefers a liquid preparation, use co-danthrusate suspension; 5 ml is equivalent to I capsule.

If necessary 'uncork' with suppositories, e.g. bisacodyl 10 mg and glycerine 4 g.

If suppositories are ineffective, administer a phosphate enema; possible repeat the next day

If the maximum dose of co-danthrusate is ineffective, reduce by half and add an osmotic laxative, e.g. lactulose 20–30 ml b.d.

If co-danthrusate causes abdominal cramps divide the total daily dose into smaller, more frequent doses, e.g. change from co-danthrusate 2 capsules b.d. to I capsule q.d.s. or change to an osmotic laxative, e.g. lactulose 20–40 ml o.d.–t.d.s.

Lactulose may be preferable to co-danthrusate in patients with a history of irritable bowel syndrome or of colic with other colonic stimulants, e.g. senna.

Sometimes it is appropriate to optimize a patient's existing bowel regimen, rather than change automatically to co-danthrusate.

---

a in USA, use Peri-Colace (casanthranol 30 mg + docusate sodium 100 mg) capsules instead.

In this situation, given time, it is usually possible to relieve the pain adequately, prevent the clock watching and demanding behaviour, and eventually change to an oral preparation. Even here it cannot be said that the patient is addicted. He is not demanding the opioid in order to experience its psychological effect but to be relieved from pain for a few hours.

Physical dependence develops in most patients who have taken an opioid regularly be mouth for more than 3–4 weeks. This is not a problem for dying patients because they generally continue on regular morphine until they die.

Some patients live for much longer than expected. If their pain disappears, the dose of morphine can be decreased and possibly stopped altogether in the following way

- if a patient – typically an outpatient – has been entirely painfree for 4 or more weeks, on a regular unchanged dose of morphine and remains relatively well, decrease the dose on a trial basis by 20–50%

- if the pain recurs, increase the dose back to the original level

- if the pain does not return and the patient feels well, the dose of morphine should be decreased again after another 7 days

- do *not* lengthen the intervals between doses.

35   Do patients die of morphine-induced respiratory depression?

No. This is because pain antagonizes the central depressant effects of morphine. When morphine is used in the way described in this book, clinically important respiratory depression is rarely seen. Should it occur

- reduce the dose of morphine if the patient is painfree

- consider using an opioid antagonist, e.g. naloxone 20 mcg IV every 2 min until the patient's respiratory status is satisfactory (*see* p.40); *this is rarely necessary.*

Iatrogenic overdosage and respiratory depression can occur, however, if the dose of morphine is increased automatically on chart rounds without bedside re-evaluation.

36   Are there any circumstances in which treatment with morphine has to be abandoned?

On rare occasions, yes (Table 3.3). Methadone, phenazocine or transdermal fentanyl can be substituted for morphine in these circumstances.

Table 3.3 Morphine intolerance

Type	Effects	Initial action	Comment
Gastric stasis	Epigastric fullness, flatulence, anorexia, persistent nausea	Metoclopramide 10–20 mg q4h; cisapride 10–20 mg b.d.	If the problem persists, change to an alternative opioid
Sedation	Intolerable sedation	Reduce dose of morphine; consider methylphenidate 10 mg o.d.–b.d. or switch to an alternative opioid	Sedation may be caused by other factors (see Table 3.2); stimulant rarely appropriate
Cognitive failure	Agitated delirium with hallucinations	Reduce dose of morphine and/or prescribe haloperidol 3–5 mg stat and nocte; if necessary, switch to an alternative opioid	Some patients develop intractable delirium with one opioid but not with an alternative opioid
Myoclonus	Multifocal twitching and/or jerking of limbs	Reduce dose of morphine but revert to former dose if pain recurs; consider clonazepam 0.5–2 mg stat and nocte	Unusual with typical oral doses; more common with high dose IV and spinal morphine
Hyperexcitability	Abdominal muscle spasms and symmetrical jerking of legs; whole-body allodynia and hyperalgesia manifesting as excruciating pain	Change to an alternative opioid	A rare syndrome in patients receiving IT or high dose IV morphine; occasionally seen with typical PO and SC doses

continued

Table 3.3 *continued*

Type	Effects	Initial action	Comment
Vestibular stimulation	Incapacitating movement-related nausea and vomiting	Cyclizine or dimenhydrinate or promethazine 25–50 mg q8h–q6h	Rare; try an alternative opioid or levomepromazine
Histamine release cutaneous	Pruritus	Oral antihistamine (e.g. chlorphenamine 4 mg b.d.–t.d.s.)	If the pruritus does not settle in a few days, prescribe an alternative opioid
bronchial	Bronchoconstriction → dyspnoea	IV/IM antihistamine (e.g. chlorphenamine 5–10 mg) and a bronchodilator	Rare; change to a chemically distinct opioid immediately, e.g. methadone or phenazocine

More questions about morphine

37   Why do some people need more morphine than others?

There are many reasons including

- age; older people tend to need less
- differences in pain intensity
- whether adjuvant drugs and nondrug measures are used
- pharmacokinetic differences:
  absorption
  'first pass' hepatic metabolism
  plasma halflife
  renal function
- genetic differences in patient's pain tolerance threshold (relates to CNS endorphin stores)
- acquired differences in patient's pain tolerance threshold (relates mainly to mood and morale)
- previously induced tolerance:
  needless increase in dose
  initial use of morphine by injection in excessive amounts
- previous use of strong opioids
- duration of treatment (tendency for the dose to increase as the disease progresses)
- adequacy of management of other symptoms.

38   Is oral morphine really effective?

Yes. Morphine sulphate/hydrochloride has been used in doses ranging from less than 5 mg *to more than 1200 mg* q4h. Published data show that for ordinary morphine tablets and aqueous solution

- the median maximum dose is 15–20 mg q4h
- few patients ever need more than 200 mg q4h
- patients with inadequate relief on 100 mg q4h may obtain benefit at higher doses.

Controlled trials have shown that m/r tablets are equally effective. This means that for m/r morphine, the median maximum dose is likely to be about 60 mg b.d. and few patients will need more than 600 mg b.d.

It is rarely necessary to prescribe morphine by injection because oral morphine is not working.

39 Is it necessary to give more morphine by mouth than by injection?

Yes. The dose of morphine sulphate should be doubled when converting from SC to PO, and trebled from IV to PO. In a few patients, further adjustment *up or down* may be necessary.

The much quoted sixfold conversion ratio from oral to parenteral morphine is incorrect. It relates to a single dose study and does not hold for regular administration. Giving 6 times as much morphine by mouth as by injection is likely to cause sedation and possibly respiratory depression.

40 Wouldn't injections be better?

No. Injections are *not* better, and can be uncomfortable. Regular injections tie the patient to a second person, generally a nurse, because someone else is needed to administer the medication. Likewise, SC infusions should not be used unless the patient cannot swallow or retain oral medication.

41 What are the indications for injections?

Main

- intractable vomiting
- inability to swallow
- coma.

Subsidiary

- psychological aversion to oral medication
- poor alimentary absorption (rare).

If regular injections become necessary, a *continuous SC infusion* of morphine is preferable to repeated doses. Several portable syringe drivers are available. *The dose of morphine should be halved when changing to the SC route.*

Diamorphine (di-acetylmorphine, heroin) is commonly used in the UK as the parenteral strong opioid of choice. When converting from oral morphine to *SC diamorphine*, the dose of oral morphine sulphate should be *divided by 3* to determine the dose of diamorphine hydrochloride.

If converting to hydromorphone, the dose of oral morphine should be *divided by 12* to determine the SC dose and adjusted if necessary. In some patients, transdermal fentanyl may be a better option.

42   Once on injections, is it possible to change successfully to the oral route?

Once vomiting has been relieved with parenteral anti-emetics, it is often possible to convert both analgesic and anti-emetic to the oral route.

It may be wise to convert to the oral route in stages, e.g. change the anti-emetic first, and morphine the next day if all remains under control.

43   When close to death and the patient becomes unconscious, should the morphine be discontinued?

No, for two main reasons

• unconscious patients in pain become restless

• physical dependence develops after several weeks of oral morphine therapy.

Thus, if the morphine is stopped abruptly, the patient will become restless, sweaty and might develop faecal incontinence secondary to rebound hyper-peristalsis. It takes only one quarter of the analgesic dose, however, to prevent opioid withdrawal phenomena.

44   Can morphine be given by suppository?

Yes. Suppositories of morphine sulphate are available in several strengths. They can also be made by any helpful pharmacist. The oral to rectal potency ratio is 1:1. In other words, the same amount is needed PR as PO. Suppositories are a useful alternative to injections, particularly in the home.

If administration q4h proves difficult, it is possible to give m/r morphine tablets PR q12h. Pharmacokinetic studies have demonstrated that they are equally well absorbed by this route.

45   What's so special about q4h?

Extensive clinical experience has shown that increasing the dose of morphine solution to provide relief for 4 h achieves the optimum balance between relief, practical convenience and adverse effects.

Giving more at less frequent intervals will provide comfort for a longer period, but only at the price of more troublesome adverse effects, particularly drowsiness and nausea.

Giving less at more frequent intervals simply makes the regular taking of morphine more tedious for the patient, particularly at night. Compliance is then reduced and more pain is the result.

The general rule is: *give morphine q4h regularly (or b.d. if a m/r preparation is used)*.

46   For ordinary morphine tablets and solution, are there any exceptions to the q4h rule?

Regular morphine is indicated for continuous pain but *not* for occasional pain. Other circumstances in which it may be desirable to prescribe morphine solution *less often* include

- the very old (90+)
- patients with night pain only
- patients with evening and night pain only
- patients in renal failure.

47   Is it ever necessary to give morphine more often than q4h?

Yes. Very occasionally a patient appears to metabolize morphine exceptionally fast. Increasing the dose in an attempt to prolong relief from 3 h to 4 h does little except increase adverse effects. If this is the case, the dose should be decreased again and given *q3h*.

A comparable situation may be seen with m/r morphine tablets. Here, the frequency of administration should be increased to *q8h*.

48   How can I tell if administration q3h is indicated?

The following will help you decide:

'Is the pain completely absent from one dose of medicine to the next?'

If the answer is 'No', then ask:

'Does the pain completely go but come back before your next dose is due, or does the medicine just ease the pain but never make you painfree?'

If it just eases the pain, a morphine increment is clearly required. If it goes and returns, the patient *may* be a fast metabolizer. The correct course is to increase the morphine by one or two increments and monitor both relief and adverse effects. If there is *minimal* improvement in pain relief but a considerable increase in adverse effects (drowsiness, vomiting), revert to the former smaller dose and increase the frequency to q3h.

Because q3h is more inconvenient to the patient than q4h, the first step is always to increase the dose of morphine rather than immediately to decrease the interval between doses. *It is rarely necessary to give morphine q3h.*

A comparable series of questions should be asked of patients receiving m/r tablets to decide if administration should be q8h.

The above advice is given on the assumption that the doctor is treating a morphine-responsive pain and that appropriate nondrug measures are being used. As emphasized elsewhere, attempts to obliterate morphine-resistant and movement-related pains with morphine generally result in severe adverse effects.

49   Should patients be awakened to take a dose in the middle of the night?

Theoretically yes, but in practice often no. A dose in the middle of the night is advisable if

- a patient is already taking one and has established a routine; it may be wise not to change this immediately

- the patient wakes regularly to micturate between 0100 h and 0300 h. Here it is unnecessary to attempt all night analgesic cover; the patient can take a dose when he gets up to micturate

- attempts to achieve all night relief have failed, and the patient continues to wake in pain in the second half of the night (0300–0600 h).

50 Can a dose in the middle of the night be avoided in other circumstances?

Yes. We regard it as the norm for the patient to sleep through the night without a dose at 0200 h. This has been achieved by modifying the q4h regimen to q4h during the day (0600 h, 1000 h, 1400 h, 1800 h) and a *double dose at bedtime* (2200 h). The greater potential for drowsiness when morphine is given in a large dose q8h is turned to good effect – the patient sleeps more soundly.

51 Is a double dose more dangerous?

A double dose of morphine at bedtime is perfectly safe in most patients. In the very frail and/or elderly, particularly if there is a risk that they might wake in the night disoriented or feeling drugged, it is wise to start with a 50% higher dose at bedtime, rather than a double dose.

52 What about the Brompton Cocktail?

This anachronistic mixture of morphine sulphate and cocaine in a vehicle of syrup, alcohol and chloroform water offers no advantages over a simple aqueous solution of morphine sulphate and *causes more adverse effects*. It is more nauseating (because of the syrup) and may cause a burning sensation in the throat (because of the alcohol). If a patient finds aqueous morphine unacceptably bitter, milk, fruit juice or other flavouring can be added at the time of administration. Alternatively, a proprietary preparation which includes a masking taste can be prescribed.

53 Is diamorphine (heroin) better than morphine?

By mouth, morphine and diamorphine (di-acetylmorphine, heroin) have similar actions and adverse effects. Diamorphine is effectively a prodrug of morphine; by the time it reaches the opioid receptors in the CNS it has been de-acetylated to morphine.

Box 3.B   Advice for patients wishing to drive while taking oral morphine

---

The medicines you are taking *do not* necessarily disqualify you from driving.

The speed of your reactions and general alertness, however, may be affected by your medication.

It is important that you take the following precautions, particularly if you have not driven for some weeks because of ill health

- do not drive in the dark or when conditions are bad
- do not drink alcohol during the day
- check your fitness to drive in the following way:
    choose a quiet time of the day when the light is good
    choose an area where there are several quiet roads
    take a companion (husband, wife, friend)
    drive for 10–15 min on quiet roads
    if both you and your companion are happy with your attentiveness, reactions and general ability, then it is all right to drive for short distances
- do not exhaust yourself by long journeys.

---

54   What about driving?

Most patients receiving morphine are not well enough to drive, and have no wish to do so. Some are much stronger and are continuing to work. Patients who wish to drive need specific advice (Box 3.B).

Doctors have an ethical and legal responsibility to advise patients if a disability is likely to make them a danger when driving. In many states and countries, there is an obligation on the driver to report any such disability to the licensing authority, unless relatively short term, e.g. less than 3 months. The patient can fulfil this obligation only if his doctor advises him appropriately.

In some countries, e.g. the USA, there are driving centres which can provide an objective evaluation of a person's capability to drive.

55   If morphine is prescribed more than a few weeks before the patient's death, what happens when tolerance develops?

Tolerance is not a practical problem when morphine is used regularly and prophylactically in individually optimized doses, and within the context of 'total patient care'. Many patients continue on an unchanged dose for weeks or months. In some, it is possible to reduce the dose after several weeks without any breakthrough pain. Rapid escalation of dose is not necessary when morphine is used properly.

56   Don't patients die quickly once morphine has been prescribed?

Many patients prescribed morphine are near to death and remain near to death. These will die quickly. On the other hand, many patients survive more than 4 weeks, some for more than 3 months, and others for over a year.

Whether the patient dies in a short time depends when morphine therapy is started. Circumstantial evidence suggests that many patients survive for a longer period because they are able to rest, sleep, eat more, and take a renewed interest in life.

On the other hand, giving morphine to a patient totally exhausted by unrelieved pain and insomnia, particularly if elderly, may lead to pneumonia consequent upon a combination of drowsiness and cough suppression. The risk is small when used in the way described in this book.

57   If patients have morphine at home, won't it get stolen?

I know of no patient whose morphine was stolen by intruders. There have been rare reports of misappropriation by a relative or a friend.

58   Won't patients use their morphine to commit suicide?

I know of no example of self-poisoning by a cancer patient in which morphine was the agent used. In any case, the incidence of suicide in cancer patients is only two or three times that of the general population.

59   Isn't the use of morphine tantamount to prescribing a living death?

Many doctors and nurses have a markedly negative attitude towards the medicinal use of morphine. As one doctor wrote, 'What about the inoperable cancer patient who may not die for months or a year, and yet who is suffering agonies from chronic pain? Is a doctor then justified in prescribing such drugs when he knows full well he will be sentencing his patient to a kind of living death?'

And although they might not express it so, doctors still share the view of the doctor who said, 'I try to postpone giving morphia until the very end and am best pleased if the first dose of morphia is also the last.'

These views stem from ignorance about and misunderstanding of the correct use of morphine in cancer patients with pain. Indeed, the patients who are truly sentenced to a kind of living death are the ones who are *not* prescribed adequate doses of morphine. One man had been bedbound for 2 months because of pain. His wife then found him crawling around the living room on his hands and knees searching for his gun which she had hidden for fear he would shoot himself. The subsequent correct use of morphine enabled this patient to live a far more normal life than would otherwise have been possible. The same is true for thousands of others.

60 Is oral morphine the panacea for cancer pain?

Definitely not! Oral morphine is a useful treatment without which life would be extremely uncomfortable for many patients with advanced cancer. It must be used correctly with an awareness of its limitations and with regular supervision for each patient.

61 What are the more important nondrug treatments?

- psychological support of the patient and family
- modification of the patient's way of life (for pains precipitated or exacerbated by movement)
- radiation therapy (principally for bone pain).

Nerve blocks have been replaced almost entirely by spinal analgesia with morphine, bupivacaine +/− clonidine. There are, of course, many other nondrug treatments – too many to list here.

62 When treating the cancer patient in pain, what else must I bear in mind?

The International Association for the Study of Pain defines pain as *an unpleasant sensory and emotional experience*. Because pain is a somatopsychic experience, its intensity is modified by the patient's mood and morale, and the meaning of the pain for the patient (Figure 3.1).

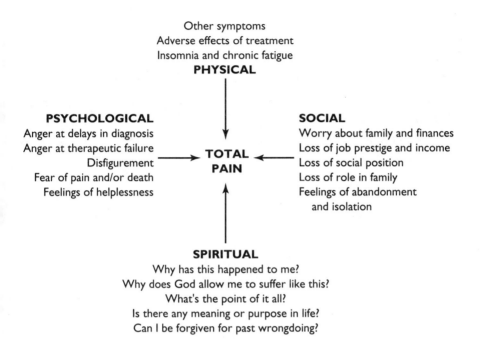

Figure 3.1   Factors influencing the perception of pain.

Those caring for the patient with cancer must be aware of the many factors which influence the patient's perception of discomfort. If a doctor is not prepared to address the many factors influencing the perception of pain, it would be wise not to prescribe morphine, but to ask a colleague who is more willing and possibly more able to look after the care of the patient.

'As the doctor–patient relationship improved, many doctors found they could reduce the drugs. As the true diagnosis of the patient's pain became clear and the patient was helped to deal with the pain of dying, there was less need for sedatives, tranquillizers, and analgesics.'   (Harte)

'No-one who hasn't time for chat knows anything about terminal care, however brilliant a clinical pharmacologist he may be.'   (Smithers)

Other important uses of morphine

63   How is morphine used to relieve dyspnoea?

Patients with dyspnoea caused by irreversible malignant chest disease often benefit from the prescription of oral morphine.

The use of morphine is aimed at reducing the *sensation* of breathlessness. Its use implies that

- reversible factors have been treated, e.g. heart failure and bronchospasm
- general guidance about coping with dyspnoea has been given.

If a resting respiratory rate of 30/min, rising to 40 or more on mild exertion, distresses and frightens the patient, it should be treated. As with pain relief, morphine should normally be given q4h to patients with dyspnoea.

Much of the benefit from morphine relates to a reduction in the futile respiratory overdrive which is commonly seen in patients with diffuse pulmonary malignant disease. This is possibly caused by the respiratory stimulant effect of multiple small areas of atelectasis.

64   What is the right dose of morphine for dyspnoea?

The dose of morphine to reduce dyspnoea tends to be smaller than those used to relieve pain

- begin with a test dose of 5–6 mg
- continue with 5–6 mg q4h, 10 mg nocte
- if there is no benefit at all and no adverse effects, increase next day to 10 mg q4h, 15–20 mg nocte
- if there is some benefit but the resting respiratory rate remains more than 24/min, increase the dose after 2–3 days and review
- consider further adjustment to morphine 15–20 mg q4h after 2–3 more days.

If a patient is already receiving morphine for pain management, the dose of morphine should be increased by 50% on a trial basis. At each stage, benefits must be weighed against adverse effects. The aim is a more relaxed patient who is not cyanosed and is mentally clear.

65 Is oral morphine of value in other forms of terminal illness?

Yes. There are at least two other situations in which morphine should be considered

- to ease the aches and discomforts of the patient who is bedbound and dying slowly; small daytime doses, e.g. 5–6 mg q4h, and a larger dose nocte, e.g. 10 mg, may make a considerable difference to the comfort of the dying

- as a cough sedative and/or night sedative in patients with motor neurone disease/amyotrophic lateral sclerosis.

Most patients with this disorder develop progressive impairment of the lower cranial nerves. This results in progressive dysarthria and dysphagia. Associated with the dysphagia is a tendency to choke unpredictably when eating or drinking, and at night as a result of aspiration of saliva. The resulting terror and anticipatory fear is a major problem in the management of terminal motor neurone disease.

Although dietary advice and explanation may help, a pharyngeal sedative is generally necessary to prevent or minimize the bouts of choking. Begin with oral morphine 5–6 mg nocte or b.d. and go on to titrate dose and frequency in the light of the initial response. Many patients need only 5–6 mg t.d.s. before meals with perhaps a larger dose nocte; a few take it q4h.

4 Psychological symptoms

Psychological problems · Anger · Anxiety
Depression · The withdrawn patient
The difficult patient · Wakeful nights
Secondary mental disorders · Delirium

Psychological problems

Patients with cancer experience psychological as well as physical symptoms. The results of a survey at a major cancer centre in the USA illustrate this point (Table 4.1). Problems are also common among patients' relatives.

Table 4.1 Common symptoms in cancer patients[1]

Physical	%	Psychological	%
Lack of energy	73	Worrying	72
Pain	63	Feeling sad	67
Drowsiness	60	Feeling nervous	62
Dry mouth	55	Difficulty sleeping	53
Nausea	45	Feeling irritable	47
Anorexia	45	Difficulty concentrating	40

Many of the psychological problems relate to actual or anticipated loss (Table 4.2). Similar psychological responses occur with losses of any kind, e.g. loss of a job, amputation, divorce, bereavement, as well as the anticipated loss of one's own life.

These phases are generally not discrete. Oscillations in the patient's feelings are common. In cancer patients, more marked responses may be seen

- at or shortly after the time of diagnosis

- at the time of the first recurrence

- at each major sign of disease progression.

Table 4.2   Psychological responses to loss[2]

Phase	Symptoms	Typical duration
Disruption	Disbelief Denial Shock/numbness Despair	< 1 week
Dysphoria	Anxiety Insomnia Anger Guilt Sadness Poor concentration Activities disrupted	Several weeks
Adaptation	Dysphoria diminishes Implications confronted New goals established Hope refocused and restored Activities resumed	Begins within 2–3 weeks

Denial

Denial is a common coping mechanism. It signifies an ability to obliterate or minimize threatening reality by ignoring it. It may be associated, however, with physiological and other nonverbal evidence of anxiety.

Most patients and relatives continue to make use of denial to a varying extent. Patients experience conflict between the wish to know the truth and the wish to avoid anxiety. Denial is one way of coping with this. Professional intervention may be needed when denial persists and interferes with

- the acceptance of treatment
- planning for the future
- relationships.

Anger, anxiety, depression

These are discussed elsewhere (*see* pp 95, 97, 100).

Paranoid states

Paranoid states may be caused by corticosteroids, biochemical disturbance, cerebral metastases or psychological factors. For example, unable to accept that he is dying, the patient believes there is a plot to kill him or the treatment is the cause of his deterioration.

Family problems

Cancer always changes family psychodynamics, either for better or for worse. Within families, there is a conflict between the wish to confide and to receive emotional and practical support on the one hand and the wish to protect others from distress, particularly children or frail parents, on the other. A conspiracy of silence is a source of tension. It blocks discussion of the future and preparation for parting. If not resolved, the bereaved often experience much regret.

Other problems

Cancer-related

e.g. impact on sexual function; difficulty in accepting a colostomy, paraplegia or the effects of cerebral secondaries

Treatment-related

e.g. adverse drug effects such as hair loss

Patients may want to share in decisions about when to stop treatment aimed at prolonging life. Fear of death may make some want to go on even when adverse effects are severe and the chance of improvement is minimal. Others may wish to opt for a shorter life of better quality when doctors are advocating more aggressive measures.

Concurrent

e.g. a bereavement or a pre-existing psychiatric illness

Management

Psychological problems are easily overlooked by doctors and nurses. Open questions, e.g. 'How are you feeling?' and 'How are you coping?' may facilitate the expression of negative emotion.

Some psychological problems can be prevented by

- good staff–patient communication, giving information according to individual need. Unfortunately, staff may not give as much information as patients and families need, even when asked directly

- good staff–patient relationships, with continuity of care
- allowing patients to have some control over the management of their illness.

There is no one right way of responding and adjusting to a poor prognosis. The doctor's task is to help the patient adjust in the best way possible, given that particular patient's background – familial, cultural and spiritual. Many people have a combination of inner resources and good support from the family and others which enable them to cope without prolonged and disabling distress.

Anxiolytics and/or antidepressants are often necessary adjuncts to psychological and social measures. Appropriate treatment will enable the patient to

- have a better quality of life during the illness
- prepare for death
- retain individuality and self-respect to the end.

Anger

Anger is an uncomfortable dynamic emotion which ranges from a mild sense of irritation to uncontrollable rage. Anger is generally transient but may be prolonged or chronic.

'A person loses his temper when the emotional demands of the situation exceed the emotional resources.'

'Anger is an emotional response to the perception of an overwhelming threat.'

Anger often

- increases vigour/energy
- facilitates the expression of negative feelings
- disrupts relationships (temporarily or permanently)
- induces impulsive action
- helps a person to defend himself physically and psychologically
- instigates aggression.

If anger is displaced or projected onto the family or staff, it tends to alienate those who want to care. Anger can also interfere with the acceptance of limitations, and may stop a patient from making positive adjustments to physical disability.

If anger is suppressed, the patient may become withdrawn, unco-operative or even depressed.

Causes

Anger is a common response to the losses inherent in living with advanced cancer (and to bereavement). There are, however, many specific causes which need to be identified (Table 4.3).

Table 4.3 Selected causes of anger in patients with advanced cancer

Personality trait
Delay in diagnosis
Manner in which the patient was told the diagnosis
Part of adjustment reaction to diagnosis and prognosis
Delay in treatment
Uncommunicative doctors
Failed treatment
Feeling of unfairness about illness
Feeling let down by God
Frustration because of limitations imposed by progressive illness
Depression

Management

Anger is a normal response to bad news and may be directed at the doctor. It is important to

- listen carefully to what is being expressed
- validate the patient's feelings, e.g. 'Given what you're having to cope with, you've every right to be angry'
- remember that a period of silence can be therapeutic

- clarify the cause(s) of anger, e.g. 'Can you bear to tell me exactly what's making you so angry?'

- consider whether anger is part of a clinical depression; if this seems probable, treat accordingly (*see* p.100)

- if anger becomes prolonged/chronic, consider obtaining help from a counsellor, psychotherapist, psychiatrist or chaplain/spiritual adviser.

With time, most patients manage to reduce anger to tolerable levels but occasionally this does not happen. *Some patients die angry.*

Anxiety

Anxiety is a universally experienced unpleasant emotion (Table 4.4). It can be acute/transient or chronic/persistent. It may be remittent/variable in intensity.

Many cancer patients sleep badly, have frightening dreams or are reluctant to be left alone at night, and sometimes during the day as well. These symptoms all suggest heightened anxiety.

Physical symptoms are common but vary considerably between people. They include palpitations, chest pain, dyspnoea, dry mouth, dysphagia, anorexia, nausea, diarrhoea, frequency of micturition, dizziness, sweating, tremor, headache, muscle tension, fatigue, weakness of the legs.

Table 4.4 Symptoms of anxiety[3]

Core features	Key symptoms
Persistently tense and unable to relax	Poor concentration
Worry	Indecisiveness
More than normal mood variation	Insomnia
Cannot distract self or be distracted out of it	Irritability
	Sweating, tremor, nausea
	Panic attacks

Causes

There are many causes of anxiety in advanced cancer (Table 4.5).

Table 4.5 Causes of heightened anxiety in advanced cancer

Situational causes	*Caused by drugs*
Adjustment disorder (i.e. an exaggerated reaction)	Corticosteroids
	Neuroleptics → akathisia (*see* p.356)
Fear of hospital, chemotherapy, radiotherapy	Drug-induced hallucinations
	benzodiazepines
Worry about family and finances	opioids
Persecutory fantasies, conscious and unconscious	Withdrawal from
	benzodiazepines
	alcohol
Organic causes	*Causes relating to a patient's inner world*
Severe pain	Thoughts about the past, e.g. wasted
Insomnia	opportunities, guilt
Weakness	Thoughts about the future
Nausea	fear of pain
Dyspnoea	fear of incontinence
Hypoglycaemia	fear of mental impairment
Brain tumour	fear of loss of independence
Secondary mental disorders (*see* p.109)	Thoughts about after death
Psychiatric causes	
Panic attacks	
Phobias	
Depression	
Delirium (50% experience anxiety)	

Evaluation

The belief that an anxious patient has the right to be anxious because he has cancer is a common obstacle to evaluation and appropriate treatment.

Review medication and consider organic causes. The main diagnostic aid is *skilled dialogue* with the patient and close relative(s).

Management

General measures

Management depends on cause

- relieve pain and other distressing symptoms
- facilitate the airing and sharing of worries and fears; 'a trouble shared is a trouble halved'
- correct misconceptions
- develop a strategy for coping with uncertainty.[4]

Drugs

These should be used together with psychological support

- benzodiazepine:
  night sedative (see p.109)
  diazepam (see p.340)
- antidepressant:
  if anxiety-depression (see p.100)
  if panic attacks
- neuroleptics:
  if delirium
  if made worse by benzodiazepines.

Psychological therapies

These are beyond the scope of this book but include a wide range of approaches (Table 4.6). They are also used in pain management, particularly when anxiety is a concurrent feature.

Table 4.6   Psychological methods for managing anxiety and/or pain

Distraction	Behavioural therapy
Creative activity	Cognitive therapy
Art therapy	Psychodynamic therapies, e.g.
Imagery	psycho-analysis
	psychodrama
Relaxation	person-centred therapy
	transactional analysis
Music therapy	family therapy
Biofeedback	Asian psychotherapies
	multimodal therapy
Hypnosis	

Depression

A major depressive illness occurs in about 5–10% of patients with advanced cancer.[5] Another 10–20% will have some depressive symptoms. Untreated depression

- intensifies other symptoms

- leads to social withdrawal

- prevents the patient from completing 'unfinished business'.

It is important to identify depression particularly because conventional treatment leads to a good response in > 80% of cases. Evidence suggests that many cases are not diagnosed. Reasons for this include

- low mood ignored by doctors and nurses because it is considered 'understandable' or 'reactive'

- diurnal variation – when seen by the doctor the patient may be feeling better than earlier in the day

- smiling depression – social skills mask the depressed mood

- somatization – the depression is expressed through one or more physical symptoms, e.g. pain

- depression masked by concomitant symptoms of anxiety

• depression manifests as a worsening of a personality trait, e.g. attention-seeking.

Risk factors

There are many risk factors predisposing to depression in advanced cancer (Table 4.7).

Table 4.7   Risk factors for depression

Biological predisposition	Loss of independence
Past history of depression	Spiritual difficulties
Inability to express emotions	Persistent pain
Conspiracy of silence	Hypercalcaemia
Lack of supportive/confiding relationship	Drugs
Recent bereavement(s)	antihypertensives
	benzodiazepines
Mutilation	corticosteroids
	cytotoxics
Threat of death	neuroleptics

Diagnosis

A major difficulty in diagnosis is that the somatic symptoms of depression are also common symptoms of cancer, namely

• anorexia

• weight loss

• constipation

• sleep disturbance

• loss of libido.

Despite its limitations in patients with advanced cancer,[6] the Hospital Anxiety and Depression (HAD) Scale is still a convenient screening tool because it excludes most of the somatic symptoms of depression which are also symptoms of advanced cancer.[5] One the other hand, because essentially it measures anhedonia (loss of pleasure in life), it cannot distinguish between a depressive illness and profound sadness. It is necessary, therefore, not only to have a checklist for possible depressive symptoms (Table 4.8) but also a list of features which help to distinguish depression from sadness (Table 4.9).

Table 4.8   Diagnostic criteria of depression in advanced cancer[3]

1   Low mood which the patient recognizes as being qualitatively and quantitatively different from normal variations in mood and from previous periods of unhappiness.
2   Depression of mood which persists for at least 2 weeks and occupies over 50% of each day.
3   Patient not able to banish the depression or be distracted out of it.
4   At least four other symptoms of depression which cannot be attributed to the physical disease: sleep disturbance – repeated waking or early morning waking loss of weight and appetite impaired concentration problems in making decisions feelings of hopelessness feelings of irritability feelings of guilt or unworthiness inability to enjoy life loss of interest increasing difficulty with daily chores.

Although more common than in the general population, suicide in cancer is still rare. Risk factors for suicide include depression, other psychiatric disorders, recent bereavement, social isolation, fears of serious physical deformity or suffering, and severe unrelieved symptoms.

Physical factors include a range of medical conditions including Huntington's chorea, AIDS, multiple sclerosis, systemic lupus erythematosus, spinal cord injury, and cancer (particularly of the head and neck).[7] Some cancers, however, do not carry an increased risk, namely nonHodgkin lymphoma, cancer of cervix uteri and cancer of the prostate. There is no additional risk in rheumatoid arthritis and motor neurone disease.[7]

Table 4.9 Distinguishing a depressive illness from sadness[8]

Features of both	Features suggesting depression
Depressed mood	Low mood which is different
Tearfulness	Loss of all emotion
Anxiety	Not distractable but diurnal variation
Suicidal ideas	Irritability
Decreased sleep	Physical anxiety
Tiredness	(sweating, tremor, panic attacks)
Decreased concentration	Hopelessness
	(particularly with regard to family and friends)
Loss of interest	Guilt
Anorexia	Intractable pain
	Suicide attempts
	Requests for euthanasia

Management

Explanation

The nature of the explanation will vary according to the patient's physical and psychological state. Patients are often helped by being told that depression is not shameful. For example:

'It seems to me that you've developed a depressive illness. [*pause*] Being physically ill is hard work and emotionally exhausting. The continued stress depletes certain chemicals in the brain which result in depression. [*pause*] Antidepressants are tablets which help the brain replenish the depleted chemicals...'

Social integration

Attendance at a palliative care day centre is helpful for patients who are isolated at home because of weakness and/or other debilitating symptoms. A day centre provides

• social interaction

- psychological support
- medical supervision.

Drugs

The choice of antidepressant is dictated partly by cost, availability and fashion but also by a desire to keep adverse effects to a minimum. For example, amitriptyline is cheap and widely available but causes more adverse effects than dothiepin and desipramine. The current vogue for SSRIs is based on an improved adverse effects profile. Sometimes, however, the choice of antidepressant is influenced by the type of depression, e.g. retarded rather than agitated (see p.349).

The withdrawn patient

Some patients seem to be psychologically inaccessible. Although this may not be unhealthy (i.e. detrimental to the patient), there are times when the patient's facial expression and behaviour suggest considerable underlying psychological distress.

Causes

These fall into several categories (Table 4.10). Sometimes there may be two or more concurrent causal factors.

Management

Management depends on the cause. If a psychological cause seems likely, try to find a 'window' in the patient's protective shell in order to help him acknowledge the problem and begin to move forward to a healthier/more comfortable frame of mind. Good communication skills are essential to achieve this

- acknowledge *your* difficulty, e.g. 'We seem to be finding it difficult to get into conversation'
- offer the patient an invitation which he can accept or reject, e.g. 'Can you tell me why you are finding it difficult to talk to me about things?'

Table 4.10   Differential diagnosis of the withdrawn patient[9]

Personality	
Pathological	
Brain tumour(s)	
Cerebrovascular disease	
Secondary mental disorders (*see* p.109)	
Concurrent illness, e.g. hypothyroidism	
Pharmacological	
Oversedation	
Tardive dyskinesia (*see* p.357)	
Psychological	
Anger	
Collusion	} 'no point in talking about my feelings'
Distrust	
Fear	'too painful'
Guilt	} 'too embarrassed'
Shame	
Psychiatric	
Depression	'no point in talking about my feelings'
Paranoia	'too dangerous'

- if the patient then gives a clue as to the reason for the reticence, this should be gently but firmly followed up, e.g. 'Exactly what are you frightened of? Can you bear to tell me about it?'

- it is important to establish the frequency and intensity of any mood disturbance in case the patient is psychiatrically ill rather than just psychologically disturbed

- ask for specialist help if you feel you are getting nowhere.

The difficult patient

It is not possible to be equally positive about all patients. Some patients we find difficult. It is important to remember that the problem is *ours* and not the patient's (although it may be a joint problem). Thus it is better to say, 'I find Mrs Brown difficult to look after' and not, 'Mrs Brown is difficult'.

Causes

There are many reasons why a patient may be difficult to care for (Table 4.11). The difficulties elicit feelings of impotence and inadequacy in us. We feel we have failed; we have come to the end of our therapeutic resources.

Table 4.11   Reasons why a patient can be difficult to care for

Patients and/or relatives perceived as	*Patient's symptoms*
Unpleasant	Gross disfigurement
Seductive	Malodour
Ungrateful	Poor response to symptom management
Critical	Somatization
Antagonistic	
Demanding	*Transference and countertransference*
Manipulative	*reactions*
Overdependent	
Patient's behaviour	
Withdrawn	
Psychologically volatile, angry	
Depressed	

Management

Acknowledge your difficulty with the rest of the team.

Explore reasons why the patient seems difficult.

Consider your own transference and countertransference reactions, i.e. feelings evoked by certain behaviours or personality traits in the patient because of your past personal experiences – or the reverse, i.e. your behaviour or personality evoking feelings in the patient – with both parties sensing the 'vibes' and reacting to them.

Agree on a management plan as a team and record it in the notes; include revised goals.

Devise a strategy regarding the time to be spent with the patient and the family.

Accept that some problems cannot be solved.

'Slowly, I learn about the importance of powerlessness.

I experience it in my own life and I live with it in my work.

The secret is not to be afraid of it – not to run away.

The dying know we are not God.

All they ask is that we do not desert them.'[10]

Wakeful nights

Some patients catnap during the day so much that they do not sleep well at night. If this is the case it is important to determine whether being awake for part or much of the night is a problem for the patient. Or is concern about wakeful nights a problem for just the family or carers?

If the patient is not sleeping for most of the night, the situation needs to be evaluated – there may be an easily reversible cause (Table 4.12).

Table 4.12   Causes of wakeful nights in advanced cancer

Physiological causes	Caused by unrelieved symptoms
Wakeful stimuli	Pain
light	Dyspnoea
noise	Vomiting
urinary frequency	Incontinence
Sleep during daytime	Diarrhoea
long siesta	Pruritus
catnaps	Restless legs
sedative drugs	
Normal old age	*Caused by drugs*
Psychological causes	Diuretics
	Corticosteroids
Anxiety (*see* p.97)	Caffeine
Depression (*see* p.100)	Sympathomimetics
Fear of dying in sleep	Night sedative withdrawal
	Benzodiazepines (if short acting may
	lead to rebound anxiety)
	Alcohol (may cause rebound wakefulness)

Management

Explanation

Treat primary cause

- relieve disturbing symptoms
- if night pain, consider increasing 2200 h morphine to *treble* the daytime q4h dose.

Nondrug measures

- change mattress/bed if not comfortable
- facilitate expression of anxieties and fears
- increase daytime activity
- reduce light and noise at night
- hot drink at bedtime
- soothing music
- relaxation therapy/tape
- brief psychotherapy (i.e. a few sessions only).

Drugs

Modify content and timing of existing drug regimen

- corticosteroids – give as single morning dose
- anxiolytics – if receiving diazepam in daytime, convert to a single dose at 2200 h
- diuretics – use a fast acting diuretic, e.g. bumetanide, furosemide
- increase bedtime dose of morphine from double to treble daytime q4h dose (*see* p.32) or supplement bedtime m/r morphine with ordinary morphine tablets or solution.

Prescribe one or more of the following

- a night sedative (*see* p.109)
- a tricyclic drug if the patient is depressed or wakes early (*see* p.349)
- haloperidol 3–5 mg nocte, particularly if unpleasant dreams

- thioridazine or chlorpromazine 50–200 mg if haloperidol fails
- levomepromazine 50–200 mg if all else fails.

Choice of night sedative[11]

- temazepam 10–40 mg, occasionally 60 mg, is widely used (halflife 8–15 h); although most preparations achieve a peak plasma concentration in 30–60 min, some hard capsules take 2–3 h
- zopiclone 3.75–15 mg (halflife 5–6 h)
- zolpidem 5–10 mg (halflife 2 h)
- chloral hydrate 500–2000 mg; no longer widely used in the UK
- chlormethiazole 500–1500 mg; useful in the very elderly who do not settle on more usual night sedatives or haloperidol.

Zopiclone and zolpidem are nonbenzodiazepines which act on the same receptors as benzodiazepines; useful in patients who feel drugged the morning after taking temazepam. Zolpidem has the added advantage of improving symptom relief in about half of the patients with Parkinson's disease.[12]

Secondary mental disorders

These are mental disorders which are secondary to organic disease or related to chemical substances (drugs, alcohol) or both (synonym: organic mental disorders).

Secondary mental disorders are classified mainly on the basis of their key features (Table 4.13). All secondary mental disorders may be seen in patients with advanced cancer.

Table 4.13 Secondary mental disorders

Delirium	Delusional disorder
Dementia	Personality change
Amnestic disorder	Intoxication
Anxiety disorder	Withdrawal state
Mood disorder	Psychosis
Hallucinosis	

Delirium (synonyms: acute brain syndrome, acute confusional state), dementia (synonym: chronic brain syndrome) and secondary amnestic disorder are all characterized by cognitive impairment. The word confusion is often used of all three conditions. Note that

- sometimes dementia is compounded by delirium
- dementia is not generally associated with drowsiness
- some patients with cancer appear to develop dementia rapidly – and this may cause difficulty in diagnosis (Table 4.14).

Patients with cognitive impairment have identifiable cognitive defects if tested formally using, for example, the Mini-Mental State Examination.

Patients manifesting the following are sometimes misdiagnosed as confused

- not taking in what is said:
    deaf

Table 4.14 Comparison of global cognitive impairment disorders

Delirium		Dementia	
Acute		Chronic	
Often remitting and reversible		Usually progressive and irreversible	
Mental clouding (information not taken in)		Brain damage (information not retained)	
+	Poor concentration	+	
+	Impaired short term memory	+	
+	Disorientation	+	
+	Living in the past	+	
+	Misinterpretations	+	
++	Hallucinations	+	
+	Delusions	+	
Speech rambling and incoherent		Speech stereotyped and limited	
Often diurnal variation		Constant (in later stages)	
Often aware and anxious		Unaware and unconcerned (in later stages)	

anxious
too ill to concentrate

- muddled speech:
poor concentration
nominal dysphasia.

It is also important to identify hypnagogic (when going to sleep) and hypno-pompic (when waking up) hallucinations as these are normal phenomena, although more common in ill patients receiving sedative drugs.

Causes

Dementia is generally caused by Alzheimer's disease or cerebral athero-sclerosis; occasionally it is paraneoplastic. The causes of other secondary mental disorders are

- drugs

- biochemical derangement

- organ failure

- brain tumours

- paraneoplastic.

Delirium

Delirium (synonym: acute confusional state) is associated with mental clouding. This leads to a disturbance of comprehension and bewilderment. Manifestations include

- poor concentration

- impairment of short term memory

- disorientation

- misinterpretations

- paranoid ideas

- hallucinations

- rambling incoherent speech

- restlessness
- noisy/aggressive behaviour.

There may be associated drowsiness. Psychomotor activity may be increased or decreased. Increased activity may be associated with overactivity of the autonomic nervous system, i.e. facial flushing, dilated pupils, injected conjunctivae, tachycardia and sweating. Delirium is precipitated or exacerbated by many factors (Table 4.15).

Table 4.15 Precipitating factors for delirium in advanced cancer

Change of environment	Pain

Unfamiliar excessive stimuli
  too hot
  too cold
  wet bed
  crumbs in bed
  creases in sheets
	Constipation

	Urinary retention
	Infection
	Dehydration
Anxiety	Withdrawal state
Depression	alcohol nicotine
Fatigue	psychotropic drugs
	Vitamin deficiency

Management

Hallucinations, nightmares and misinterpretations represent a failure in the patient's coping mechanisms, and reflect fears and anxieties. Their content should be explored with the patient.

Explanation

- stress to both the patient and the relatives that the patient is not going mad, and there is a physical cause
- stress that there are generally lucid intervals.

Treat reversible causes

In patients suspected of having alcohol withdrawal, IV chlormethiazole 0.8% is the treatment of choice

- initially 5–15 ml (40–120 mg)/min, up to 100 ml (800 mg)/min
- continue with 0.5–1 ml (4–8 mg)/min according to response
- close supervision is necessary because the patient may lapse into deep coma, necessitating a reduction in the rate of infusion.

If the patient's agitation prevents setting up an IV infusion, give amobarbital 250 mg IM stat. This usually acts within 1–2 min and the effect lasts 1–2 h.

If nicotine withdrawal is suspected, encourage smoking or administer a medicinal nicotine product

- Nicorrette nasal spray, containing nicotine 500 mcg/metered spray
- transdermal nicotine patches, 11 mg and 22 mg in 24 h.

The cost of the transdermal patches is not covered by the National Health Service in the UK.

Nondrug measures

- continue to treat the patient with courtesy and respect
- restraints should never be used
- bed rails should be avoided – they can be dangerous
- patient should be allowed to walk about accompanied
- allay fear and suspicion, and reduce misinterpretations by:
  use of night light
  not changing the position of the patient's bed
  explaining every procedure and event in detail
  the presence of a family member or close friend.

Drugs

Generally use drugs only if symptoms are marked, persistent and cause distress to the patient and/or family. Review sooner rather than later if a sedative drug is prescribed because symptoms may be exacerbated.

Consider

- reduction in medication
- oxygen if cyanosed
- dexamethasone if cerebral tumour (see p.315)
- haloperidol 1.5–5 mg PO or SC if agitated, hallucinating or paranoid.

The initial dose of haloperidol depends on previous medication, weight, age and severity of symptoms. Subsequent doses depend on the initial response; maintenance doses are generally adequate.

Terminal distress

This is often associated with delirium and may need haloperidol 10–30 mg/ 24 h and/or midazolam 10–60 mg/24 h by continuous SC infusion to control it (see p.308).

Levomepromazine 25–50 mg stat and 50–200 mg/24 h should be substituted for haloperidol if the patient remains agitated despite the combined use of haloperidol and midazolam. Alternatively, SC phenobarbital 100–200 mg stat and 800–1600 mg/24 h can be given instead of both haloperidol and midazolam.

References

1   Portenoy R et al. (1994) The Memorial symptom assessment scale: an instrument for the evaluation of symptom prevalence, characteristics and distress. European Journal of Cancer. **30A**: 1326–1336.
2   Massie MJ and Holland JC (1989) Overview of normal reactions and prevalence of psychiatric disorders. In: JC Holland and JH Rowland (eds) Handbook of Psycho-oncology. Oxford University Press, Oxford. pp 273–282.
3   Faulkner A and Maguire P (1994) Talking to cancer patients and their relatives. Oxford Medical Publications, Oxford.
4   Twycross R (1997) Introducing Palliative Care. (2nd edn) Radcliffe Medical Press, Oxford.
5   Hopwood P et al. (1991) Psychiatric morbidity in patients with advanced cancer of the breast: prevalence measured by two self-rating questionnaires. British Journal of Cancer. **64**: 349–352.
6   Faull CM et al. (1993) The hospital anxiety and depression (HAD) scale: its validity in patients with terminal malignant disease. Paper presented at the Palliative Care Research Forum, London.

7 Harris EC and Barraclough BM (1994) Suicide as an outcome for medical disorders. *Medicine (Baltimore).* **73**: 281–296.
8 Casey P (1994) Lecture at Annual Clinical Meeting of the Association of Palliative Medicine of Britain and Ireland, Dublin.
9 Maguire P *et al.* (1993) Handling the withdrawn patient – a flow diagram. *Palliative Medicine.* **7**: 333–338.
10 Cassidy S (1988) *Sharing the darkness.* Darton, Longman and Todd, London. pp 61–64.
11 Ashton CH (1997) Management of insomnia. *Prescribers' Journal.* **37**: 1–10.
12 Daniele A *et al.* (1997) Zolpidem in Parkinson's disease. *Lancet.* **349**: 1222–1223.

5 Neurological symptoms

Weakness · Lambert-Eaton myasthenic syndrome (LEMS)
Spinal cord compression · Patulous Eustachian tube
Cramp · Myoclonus · Grand mal convulsions
Stopping dexamethasone in patients with
intracranial malignancy

Weakness

Localized

Localized weakness may be caused by

- cerebral neoplasm – monoparesis, hemiparesis
- spinal cord compression – generally bilateral (*see* p.120)
- peripheral nerve lesions, e.g.
    brachial plexus lesion
    Pancoast's tumour
    axillary recurrence
    lumbosacral plexus lesion
    lateral popliteal nerve palsy
- proximal limb muscle weakness, e.g.
    corticosteroid myopathy (*see* p.318)
    paraneoplastic myopathy and/or neuropathy
    paraneoplastic polymyositis
    Lambert-Eaton myasthenic syndrome (*see* p.118).

Peripheral neuropathy secondary to diabetes or vitamin B_{12} deficiency is occasionally seen in advanced cancer. Correction of hyperglycaemia or vitamin deficiency prevents further deterioration but improvement takes time. Corrective measures are unnecessary in patients close to death.

Generalized

Generalized progressive weakness may mean that the patient is close to death. Other possibilities should be considered (Table 5.1).

Table 5.1   Causes of generalized weakness in advanced cancer

Causes	Treatment possibilities
Caused by cancer	
Progression of disease	Modify pattern of life
Anaemia	Haematinics, blood transfusion?
Hypercalcaemia	(*see* p.132)
Hypo-adrenalism	
Neuropathy	Corticosteroid
Myopathy	
Depression	Antidepressant
Caused by treatment	
Surgery	
Chemotherapy	Supervised rehabilitation
Radiation	
Drugs	
diuretics	
antihypertensives	Reduce or discontinue medication
oral hypoglycaemics	
Hypokalaemia	Potassium supplements
Related to cancer and/or debility	
Insomnia	Night sedative
Exhaustion	Rest
Prolonged bedrest	
pain	Relieve causal symptom
dyspnoea	Physiotherapy
malaise	
Infection	Antibiotic
Dehydration	Hydration
Malnutrition	Dietary advice (*see* p.168)

Management

- when weakness relates to an easily correctable cause, appropriate measures should be taken (Table 5.1)

- if weakness relates mainly to disease progression, consider a 1 week trial of corticosteroids, e.g. dexamethasone 4 mg o.d. or prednisolone 20–30 mg o.d.

- anaemia may respond to iron supplements if related to blood loss; anaemia of chronic disease does not respond to haematinics

- as the patient becomes more debilitated, the benefit of blood transfusion becomes less; treat the patient and not the haemoglobin level (*see* p.239)

- IV hyperalimentation is not indicated for weakness; it only occasionally leads to weight gain but weakness persists.

Lambert-Eaton myasthenic syndrome (LEMS)

Description

LEMS is a paraneoplastic disorder of neuromuscular transmission which occurs in 3% of patients with small cell lung cancer and occasionally with other cancers, e.g. nonsmall cell lung, breast and lymphoma.[1] LEMS is distinct from the neuropathy and myopathy which is common in lung cancer patients who have lost ≥ 15% of their body weight, i.e. a concomitant of the cachexia-anorexia syndrome.

Pathogenesis

LEMS is a paraneoplastic syndrome in which there is a presynaptic deficit in neuromuscular transmission. This is caused by a reduction in the amount of acetylcholine released on arrival of nerve impulses at the motor nerve terminal. Neurological paraneoplastic syndromes in small cell lung cancer often occur concurrently.[1] Thus, LEMS may occur with one or more of the following

- sensory neuropathy

- cerebellar degeneration

- limbic encephalopathy

- myelopathy

- visual failure.

LEMS is associated with auto-immunity. Antibodies against small cell lung cancer sometimes are crossreactive against the voltage-gated calcium-channel, an important component of the neuromuscular junction. Small cell lung cancer is thought by some to be derived from neural crest tissue, and this is thought to explain the crossreactivity with other neural tissues and the association with so many paraneoplastic neurological syndromes.

Clinical features

Symptoms

*   proximal muscle weakness:
    always present in the legs (and the presenting symptom in over 50%)
    seen in the arms in about 25% of cases
    onset generally insidious but can be abrupt
    often worse after exercise

*   diplopia (usually transient)

*   dysarthria, dysphonia, dysphagia (i.e. bulbar symptoms)

*   dry mouth (75%)

*   erectile impotence

*   constipation.

Signs

*   rolling or waddling gait associated with truncal and proximal weakness

*   transient augmentation of strength during first few seconds of muscular contractions

*   tendon reflexes are diminished or absent at rest but re-appear or increase after sustained (15 second) muscular contraction; *this is pathognomonic of a presynaptic neuromuscular transmission deficit*

*   ptosis may be present

*   strabismus is uncommon (in contrast to myasthenia gravis).

Diagnosis

LEMS generally manifests in otherwise asymptomatic small cell lung cancer patients. Patients with LEMS must therefore be investigated for lung cancer. The diagnosis of LEMS is confirmed by electrophysiological tests.[2] In > 90% of patients there is a positive assay for antibodies against the voltage-gated calcium-channel.[3]

Patients with LEMS generally feel stronger if given edrophonium 10 mg IM/IV. Edrophonium is an anticholinesterase with a duration of action of about 5 min. A negative result does not exclude the diagnosis and a positive result is also seen in myasthenia gravis.

Management

Successful anticancer treatment is often accompanied by improvement of the neurological symptoms.

Unlike other neurological paraneoplastic syndromes, LEMS generally responds to

- immunosuppression
- enhanced neuromuscular transmission.

Immunosuppression

- prednisolone 60 mg o.d. or more
- azathioprine 100–150 mg o.d.
- IV immunoglobulin 400 mg/kg for 5 days[4] ⎫ lead to improvement within 2 weeks
- plasma exchange ⎭ which lasts for up to 6 weeks.

It is possible that some cachectic patients who benefit from corticosteroids may have an immune-mediated paraneoplastic syndrome.

Enhanced neuromuscular transmission

- an anticholinesterase will enhance neuromuscular transmission, e.g. pyridostigmine 60–120 mg q4h
- 3,4-diaminopyridine (DAP) inhibits potassium flux out of neurones and thereby prolongs acetylcholine release which enhances neuromuscular transmission. DAP 10 mg q.d.s. is prescribed in the UK on a named patient basis, increasing up to 20 mg q.d.s.[1] Most patients experience dose-related paraesthesiae in association with periods of increased strength. The effects of an anticholinesterase and DAP are additive.

Spinal cord compression

Incidence

Occurs in 3% of patients with advanced cancer.

Compression occurs at more than one level in 20% of cases.

Cancers of the breast, bronchus and prostate account for 40%.

Most others are associated with

- renal cell cancer
- lymphoma
- myeloma
- melanoma
- sarcoma
- head and neck cancer.

Level of compression

- cervical 10%
- thoracic 70%
- lumbar 20%.[5]

Below the level of L2, compression is of the cauda equina, i.e. peripheral nerves and not the spinal cord.

Mechanism of compression

Spinal cord compression is caused by

- metastatic spread to a vertebral body or pedicle 85%
- tumour extension through intervertebral foramina (notably lymphoma) 10%
- intramedullary primary 4%
- haematogenous dissemination → epidural space 1%.

Presentation

- pain   > 90%
- weakness   > 75%
- sensory level   > 50%
- sphincter dysfunction   > 40%.

The patient may be unaware of sensory loss until examined, particularly if this is confined to the sacrum or perineum.

Pain generally predates other symptoms and signs of cord compression by several weeks or months. Pain may be caused by

- vertebral metastasis
- root compression
- compression of the long tracts of the spinal cord (funicular pain).

Radicular and funicular pains are often exacerbated by neck flexion or straight leg raising, and by coughing, sneezing or straining. Funicular pain is generally less sharp than radicular pain, has a more diffuse distribution (like a cuff or garter around thighs, knees or calves) and is sometimes described as a cold unpleasant sensation.

Diagnosis

- history and clinical findings
- a plain radiograph shows vertebral metastasis/collapse at the appropriate level in 80%
- a bone scan does not often yield additional information
- MRI is the investigation of choice
- CT with myelography may be helpful if MRI is not available.

Management

Patients with paraparesis do better than those who are totally paraplegic. Recovery is more likely after lesions of the cauda equina. Loss of sphincter function is a bad prognostic sign.

Rapid onset complete paraplegia (over 24–36 h) has a poor prognosis; it is almost always caused by infarction of the spinal cord secondary to tumour compression and thrombosis of a spinal artery.

The main therapeutic options are

- corticosteroids
- radiotherapy.

These act in different ways and generally should be given concurrently. Corticosteroids often bring about an early improvement and relief of pain; this relates to a reduction in peritumour inflammation. Radiotherapy brings about improvement by tumour reduction; this takes longer.

Dexamethasone is given in high doses initially. Regimens vary, e.g.

- 12 mg PO stat; 24 mg PO o.d. for 3 days
- 100 mg IV stat; 24 mg PO q.d.s. for 3 days.

Dexamethasone is rapidly reduced to 12–16 mg o.d., after which reductions are made according to the rate and completeness of response. If there is a good result, it is generally possible to stop dexamethasone.

Surgery is only occasionally indicated. Consider if

- neurological deterioration despite radiotherapy and high dose dexamethasone
- solitary vertebral metastasis
- diagnosis in doubt.

Laminectomy may well lead to further deterioration because in most cases the cord compression is anterior. In this circumstance, laminectomy is likely to exacerbate spinal instability and cord injury. Vertebral body resection with anterior spinal stabilization is generally the operation of choice.[6]

Patulous Eustachian tube

Description

The Eustachian tube is normally closed and opens only temporarily during swallowing. When the tube is patulous (i.e. remains open), free passage of air and sound occurs between the nasopharynx and the middle ear. The Eustachian tube becomes patulous particularly in pregnant women and in association with a rapid marked loss of weight. It is often misdiagnosed as serous otitis media.

Clinical features

Symptoms

Symptoms are either continuous or intermittent, and vary from a minor annoyance to a major cause of distress

- a feeling of aural fullness/pressure, generally interpreted as a blocked ear which is not relieved by swallowing
- blowing sound in ear(s) synchronous with breathing
- crackling sound when chewing
- voice sounds excessively loud and hollow, resembling an echo (autophony)
- postural variation; symptoms often diminish or disappear when patient is supine.

Signs

Auroscopy generally shows movement of the tympanic membrane synchronous with nasal inspiration and expiration.

Management

Symptoms are generally not severe and explanation is adequate. Patients benefit by discovering that in certain positions the symptoms remit, notably when supine. A sharp forceful sniff may also bring temporary relief. Other options include

- nasal drops containing hydrochloric acid, chlorbutanol, benzyl alcohol and propylene glycol[7]
- intratubal injection of:
    atropine
    liquid paraffin
    gelatine sponge
    Teflon
- insertion of a grommet (ventilating tube) in the tympanic membrane under local anaesthetic by ENT specialist using an operating microscope.

A grommet permits any air going up the Eustachian tube to escape externally instead of causing flapping of the tympanic membrane which is mainly responsible for the annoying auditory discomfort linked to breathing.

Cramp

Description

Cramp is a painful muscle spasm lasting from a few seconds to many hours or days. Some authorities, however, limit the duration of a cramp to a maximum of 10 minutes, and refer to pain lasting longer than this as painful muscle stiffness.[8]

Physiology

Cramp can be induced by nerve stimulation distal to a nerve block.[9] This suggests that cramp originates within the intramuscular motor nerve terminals. It has been postulated that in exercise, for example, unmyelinated nerve terminals are exposed to excitatory chemicals in the extracellular space of muscle and to metabolites produced by the exercising muscle. The same nerve terminals may also be excited if mechanically deformed when the muscle is maximally shortened. Cramp is also associated with acute fluid loss, for example by diuresis, sweating, diarrhoea or renal dialysis. This may relate to the mechanical effect of a contracted extracellular space on the nerve terminals.

Cramp is also associated with neural dysfunction and injury.[10] In this circumstance, neural hyperexcitability may impact peripherally on the intramuscular nerve terminals. Questions remain, however, as to why cramp does not occur more often in exercise or secondary to neural dysfunction.

Causes

Cramp is a universal experience. It occurs most commonly in a single muscle in the calf or foot. Cramp is also common in muscles close to a painful bone metastasis, particularly when movement precipitates or exacerbates pain.

Cramp may be caused by drugs (Table 5.2). Although cisplatin may cause cramp secondary to hypomagnesaemia, most cases of chemotherapy-related cramp occur in association with drug-induced peripheral neuropathy.

In a series of 50 cancer patients with severe cramp referred to a neurological clinic, an underlying pathological condition was identified in all but nine.[10] Causes included

- meningeal metastases
- nerve compression

Table 5.2   Drug-induced cramp[11,12]

Diuretics	β_2-adrenergic agonists
Chemotherapy	salbutamol
vincristine	terbutaline
cisplatin	Amitriptyline
Hormone therapy	Amphotericin B
medroxyprogesterone acetate	
other	Cimetidine
Prednisolone	Clofibrate
Beclomethasone (by inhaler)	Lithium

- peripheral neuropathy
- polymyositis
- concurrent spinal degeneration.

In some patients, the peripheral neuropathy was secondary to diabetes mellitus. Cramp occurred in

- arms only (about 10%)
- legs only (40%)
- arms and legs (40%)
- arms, legs and trunk (10%).

Most patients suffered frequent attacks, generally of brief duration (seconds → minutes). In patients with advanced cancer, cramp in the arm(s) in particular should alert the doctor to the possibility of an underlying neurological cause.

Management

Explanation

Treat reversible causes

If feasible, causal drugs should be reduced in dose or stopped at least temporarily. If associated with a neurological condition, treatment should be directed to the underlying cause.

Physical therapy

Cramp is easier to induce in a shortened muscle and cannot be induced or sustained in a stretched muscle.[9] Stretching movements (both active and passive) are therefore an important nondrug measure. Stretching of the calf and foot muscles o.d.–b.d. is a time-honoured way of reducing the frequency and severity of nocturnal calf and foot cramps. In debilitated patients, this is best done by a physiotherapist, nurse or relative. Forced dorsiflexion of the foot for 5–10 seconds repeated for up to 5 minutes stretches both calf and foot muscles. It is an uncomfortable procedure but the nocturnal benefit generally outweighs any short term discomfort.

Some patients may be fit enough to stretch their own muscles by leaning with both hands against a wall and with one leg bent to provide stability and the other stretched back with the dorsiflexed foot firmly on the floor. Stretching is aided by 'rocking' on the dorsiflexed foot. After stretching the muscles of one leg, the positions of the two legs are reversed and the procedure repeated.

Massage and relaxation therapy are particularly important for cramp associated with myofascial trigger points (see p.18). Trigger points also benefit by injection with a local anaesthetic, e.g. lidocaine 1% or bupivacaine 0.5%. If the trigger point is secondary to muscle trauma, injection of a depot preparation of a corticosteroid (methylprednisolone or triamcinolone) may help to disrupt the trigger.

Drugs

In cancer patients with recurrent or persistent cramp, diazepam 5–10 mg nocte should be prescribed. Alternatively, baclofen 10–20 mg b.d.–t.d.s. can be tried. Both drugs work via a central inhibitory GABA mechanism which reduces muscle tone. In anxious patients, diazepam is of double benefit; it relaxes both muscles and mind.

Dantrolene acts directly on skeletal muscle and does not cause so much sedation. It is a further option and if necessary can be used in conjunction with diazepam or baclofen. The recommended starting dose is 25 mg o.d., increasing by 25 mg weekly to 100 mg q.d.s. The modal dose is 75 mg t.d.s. In palliative care it is generally necessary to titrate the dose at a faster rate because of the need for rapid relief.

For nocturnal calf or foot cramp, quinine sulphate 200 mg (or quinine bisulphate 300 mg) nocte should be considered if diazepam is ineffective.[13,14] Alternatively, quinine sulphate 200 mg may be taken with the evening meal and a further 100 mg nocte.[15] Quinine reduces the frequency of cramps and sleep disturbance but does not always reduce cramp severity.[16] The maximum benefit of quinine may not be obtained for about 4 weeks. Smoking can block the effect of quinine.[16] Quinine is an antimalarial drug and is toxic in overdose; accidental fatalities have occurred in children.

Myoclonus

Description

Myoclonus is sudden, brief, shock-like involuntary movements caused by either primary muscle contractions or secondary to CNS stimulation. Myoclonus may be

- focal (a single muscle or group of muscles), regional or multifocal (generalized)
- unilateral or bilateral (either asymmetrical or symmetrical)
- mild (twitching) or severe (jerking).

Causes

Myoclonus may be

- physiological
- primary ('essential')
- secondary to:
  neurological disorders
  metabolic disorders
  drug toxicity
  other chemical toxicity.

Secondary multifocal myoclonus is a central pre-epileptiform phenomenon and should not be ignored. It occurs mainly in moribund patients when it may relate to hypoglycaemia and/or other biochemical disturbances e.g. renal failure. It is also caused or exacerbated by drugs with anticholinergic properties and occasionally by high doses of diamorphine or morphine, or other strong opioid (see p.78).

Management

Even if longstanding, it is worth trying clonazepam 0.5 mg nocte for trouble-some primary myoclonus. If of recent onset, review medication and, if possible, reduce or stop causal or exacerbating drugs. In moribund patients, consider

- diazepam 10 mg PR and 10–20 mg PR nocte *or*
- midazolam 5 mg SC and 10 mg/24 h by SC infusion.

Adjust the dose upwards if several as needed doses are administered.

Grand mal convulsions

Emergency treatment

If a patient has a grand mal convulsion, give

- diazepam 10 mg PR and repeat after 15 and 30 min if not settled *or*
- midazolam 10 mg SC/IV and repeat after 15–20 min if not settled
- if the above fail, phenobarbital 100 mg SC *or*
- phenobarbital 100 mg in 100 ml of saline IV over 30 min.

Maintenance treatment

In moribund patients, maintenance treatment typically comprises

- diazepam 20 mg PR nocte or b.d. *or*
- midazolam 30–60 mg/24 h by continuous SC infusion *or*
- phenobarbital 200–600 mg/24 h by continuous SC infusion.

Higher doses may be used if necessary.

In relatively fit patients, the cause of the convulsion(s) needs to be invest-igated, and an appropriate oral anticonvulsant regimen started and monitored according to standard practice. When such patients are no longer able to swallow, convert to diazepam PR or midazolam by SC infusion (as above).

If some hours have elapsed since the last oral dose, it may be wise to give a stat dose of diazepam 10 mg PR or midazolam 10 mg SC. Remember

- phenytoin and sodium valproate have long plasma halflives and will be present in the patient for some time after stopping oral therapy. The continuing but diminishing effects of phenytoin and sodium valproate supplement the benzodiazepine

- phenobarbital sodium for injection is made up in 90% propylene (200 mg/ 1 ml). If given by SC infusion, it should be diluted with water. Of drugs commonly given by SC infusion, phenobarbital is miscible only with diamorphine and hyoscine.

Stopping dexamethasone in patients with intracranial malignancy

Most patients stop taking dexamethasone automatically when they become moribund and can no longer swallow. They may need diamorphine/morphine by SC infusion to prevent distressing headaches and diazepam PR/midazolam SC to prevent convulsions.

Occasionally the patient requests that the dexamethasone is stopped because of deterioration despite the continued use of dexamethasone and an unacceptable quality of life. This is a situation which tends to cause considerable staff distress.

It is probably best to reduce the dexamethasone step by step on a daily basis, because this gives the patient time to reconsider. At the same time

- increase the oral anticonvulsant medication

- prescribe additional analgesics for breakthrough headache:
    if on paracetamol, prescribe co-proxamol as needed
    if on co-proxamol, prescribe morphine 10–20 mg PO or diamorphine/
        morphine 5–10 mg as needed

- review twice a day, preferably personally:
    consider changing regular analgesics if two or more as needed doses
        have been given in the previous 24 h
    consider changing anticonvulsants to diazepam PR or midazolam SC if
        the patient becomes drowsy or finds swallowing difficult

- consider changing to diamorphine and midazolam by continuous SC infusion.

If the morphine or diamorphine causes significant respiratory depression, the elevated pCO_2 induces intracranial vasodilatation which leads to an increase in intracranial pressure and exacerbation of headache. If suspected because of restlessness, grimacing or other physical expressions of pain, it may be necessary to increase the morphine/diamorphine rapidly (possibly double or treble the dose) in order to overcome medication-exacerbated headache. In practice this is rarely necessary.

References

1   Elrington G (1992) The Lambert-Eaton myasthenic syndrome. *Palliative Medicine.* **6**: 9–17.

2   Newsom-Davis J and Murray NMF (1984) Plasma exchange and immunosuppressant drug treatment in the Lambert-Eaton Myasthenic Syndrome. *Neurology.* **34**: 480–485.

3   Motomura M *et al.* (1995) An improved diagnostic assay for Lambert-Eaton myasthenic syndrome. *Journal of Neurology, Neurosurgery and Psychiatry.* **58**: 85–87.

4   Bain PG *et al.* (1996) Effects of intravenous immunoglobulin on muscle weakness and calcium-channel autoantibodies in the Lambert-Eaton myasthenic syndrome. *Neurology.* **47**: 678–683.

5   Kramer JA (1992) Spinal cord compression in malignancy. *Palliative Medicine.* **6**: 202–211.

6   Siegal T and Siegal T (1985) Surgical decompression of anterior and posterior malignant epidural tumours compressing the spinal cord: a prospective study. *Neurosurgery.* **17**: 424–432.

7   DiBartolomeo JR (1993) Correspondence. *American Journal of Otology.* **14**: 313.

8   Jansen PHP *et al.* (1991) Clinical diagnosis of muscle cramp and muscular cramp syndromes. *European Archives of Psychiatry and Clinical Neuroscience.* **241**: 98–101.

9   Layzer RB (1994) The origin of muscle fasciculations and cramps. *Muscle and Nerve.* **17**: 1243–1249.

10 Steiner I and Siegal T (1989) Muscle cramps in cancer patients. *Cancer.* **63**: 574–577.

11 Siegal T (1991) Muscle cramps in the cancer patient: causes and treatment. *Journal of Pain and Symptom Management.* **6**: 84–91.

12 Lear J and Daniels RG (1993) Muscle cramps related to corticosteroids. *British Medical Journal.* **306**: 1169.

13 Warburton A *et al.* (1987) A quinine a day keeps the leg cramps away? *British Journal of Clinical Pharmacology.* **23**: 459–465.

14 Man-Son-Hing M and Wells G (1995) Meta-analysis of efficacy of quinine for treatment of nocturnal leg cramps in elderly people. *British Medical Journal.* **310**: 13–17.

15 Jansen PHP *et al.* (1997) Randomised controlled trial of hydroquinine in muscle cramps. *Lancet.* **349**: 528–532.

16 Connolly PS *et al.* (1992) The treatment of nocturnal leg cramps: a crossover trial of quinine vs. vitamin E. *Archives of Internal Medicine.* **152**: 1877–1880.

6 Biochemical syndromes

Hypercalcaemia
Syndrome of inappropriate antidiuresis (SIAD)

Hypercalcaemia

Hypercalcaemia is an *ionized* plasma calcium concentration above the upper limit of normal.

In most centres, the total plasma calcium concentration is measured. This includes both protein-bound and ionized calcium. If a patient is hypo-albuminaemic, the total plasma concentration may give a false impression of normality. There are several methods of 'correcting' for hypo-albuminaemia, each of which relates to the *mean normal plasma albumin* concentration for the biochemical laboratory concerned (Box 6.A).

Box 6.A Correcting plasma calcium concentrations (Oxford Radcliffe Hospital Trust)

Corrected calcium (mmol/l) = measured calcium + 0.022 × (42 − albumin (g/l))

e.g.   measured calcium = 2.45; albumin = 32

corrected calcium = 2.45 + 0.022 × 10 = 2.67 mmol/l

Incidence

All malignant disease 10–20%.

Breast, squamous lung and genito-urinary cancers and myeloma 20–40%.

Uncommon in prostate, small cell lung, gastric and large bowel cancers.

Pathogenesis

In the past, hypercalcaemia in cancer was thought to be related to metastatic bone disease and the direct release of skeletal calcium by osteolytic substances produced by the metastatic cancer. This is not so. Most patients with bone metastases remain normocalcaemic and there is no correlation between the number of bone metastases and the occurrence of hypercalcaemia. Biochemical evidence of humoral mechanisms is detectable in almost all case of hypercalcaemia in cancer.

In solid tumours, hypercalcaemia in cancer is caused by increased bone resorption induced by tumour-secreted parathyroid hormone-related protein (PTHrP). This is not detected by radio-immuno-assay for parathyroid hormone (PTH); in hypercalcaemia in cancer, plasma PTH concentrations are low or undetectable.

In myeloma, hypercalcaemia is caused by the osteoclast activating effects of cytokines such as interleukin 1, tumour necrosis factor and lymphotoxin. In lymphoma, similar factors to myeloma are responsible in some cases. In others, PTHrP is present. Some lymphomas also produce 25-vitamin D1 α-hydroxylase, the enzyme which converts 25-hydroxyvitamin D into biologically active 1,25-dihydroxyvitamin D (1,25 DHCC). This leads to increased intestinal absorption of vitamin D and an increased production of vitamin D during exposure to sunlight.

PTHrP impairs calcium excretion by the distal renal tubule, and vomiting leads to sodium loss and to sodium-linked calcium re-absorption by the proximal renal tubule. Renal impairment in myeloma is exacerbated by nephrotoxic immunoglobulin light chains.

Clinical features

Severity of symptoms is not always related to degree of hypercalcaemia. Sometimes a small elevation causes definite symptoms, and vice versa.

Mild (patient ambulatory)

- fatigue
- lethargy
- mental dullness
- weakness
- anorexia
- constipation.

Polyuria and polydipsia are not constant features.

Severe (patient increasingly incapacitated)

- nausea ⎫
- vomiting ⎬   dehydration and cardiovascular collapse
- ileus ⎭
- delirium
- drowsiness
- coma.

Severe symptoms may develop rapidly without a clearly defined prodrome.

Severe hypercalcaemia > 4 mmol/l is generally fatal if untreated because of acute renal failure and cardiac arrhythmias. Neurological symptoms and signs are seen occasionally, e.g. upper motor neurone deficits, scotomata, ataxia, fits. These can mimic cerebral secondaries. Severe dysphagia for food and fluid occasionally occurs. *Pain may be precipitated or exacerbated by hypercalcaemia.*

Diagnosis

Hypercalcaemia is seldom associated with an occult cancer. Diagnosis is based on a high level of clinical suspicion, and confirmed by appropriate blood tests; exclude alternative causes, e.g. hypervitaminosis D and milk-alkali syndrome.

In malignant hypercalcaemia there is *hypochloraemic alkalosis* whereas primary hyperparathyroidism is associated with *hyperchloraemic acidosis* because of impaired renal bicarbonate resorption. Thus, plasma chloride concentration is

- generally < 98 mmol(mEq)/l in malignant disease
- generally >103 mmol(mEq)/l in hyperparathyroidism.

Management

Stop and think! Are you justified in treating a potentially fatal complication in a moribund patient?

The following together comprise a set of indications for treating hypercalcaemia

- corrected plasma calcium concentration of > 2.8 mmol/l

- symptoms attributable to hypercalcaemia
- first episode or long interval since previous one
- previous good quality of life (in patient's opinion)
- medical judgement that treatment will achieve a durable effect (based on the results of previous treatment)
- patient willing to have IV therapy and requisite blood tests.

Median survival in one series was 5 weeks, after correction of the hypercalcaemia, ranging from < 1 week to > 1 year.[1]

Not all symptoms respond equally (Table 6.1).

Table 6.1   Response of symptoms to the treatment of hypercalcaemia[2]

Consistent	Variable
Delirium	General malaise
Mental dullness	Fatigue
Thirst	Anorexia
Polyuria	
Constipation	

Fluid replacement

- isotonic saline 3–4 l/24 h for 48 h + potassium supplements then
- 2–3 l/24 h isotonic saline + potassium supplements until adequate oral fluid intake.

Saline therapy improves hypercalcaemia by improving the glomerular filtration rate and by promoting a sodium-linked calcium diuresis. Saline alone will reduce plasma calcium concentrations by 0.2–0.4 mmol/l.

Loop diuretics

High dose loop diuretics, e.g. bumetanide 2 mg q2h or furosemide 80 mg q2h + 12 l of saline/24 h require intensive care facilities and are *not* appropriate in palliative care.

Bisphosphonates

Bisphosphonates are a group of drugs which inhibit osteoclast activity and thereby inhibit bone resorption. Bisphosphonates do not block PTHrP-mediated renal tubular re-absorption of calcium.

Because of poor alimentary absorption, bisphosphonates are generally given IV initially. Drug of choice and regimens vary (Table 6.2). Pamidronate is used at Sobell House; it is more potent than etidronate and clodronate. If corrected plasma calcium (mmol/l)

- < 3.0 give 30 mg in 250 ml saline over ≥ 30 min
- 3–3.5 give 60 mg in 250 ml saline over ≥ 60 min
- > 3.5 give 90 mg in 500 ml saline over ≥ 90 min.

Normocalcaemia is restored in < 90%; maximum effect after 5–7 days

- give 60–90 mg after 1 week if initial poor response
- repeat every 3–4 weeks depending on need.

Bisphosphonates are also used for metastatic bone pain

- IV pamidronate 90 mg every 4 weeks *prophylactically* in patients with one or more osteolytic bone metastases ≥ 1 cm in diameter;[3] *very costly*
- IV pamidronate 120 mg; if beneficial repeat as necessary every 2–4 months[4]
- clodronate is used at some centres; IV initially followed by oral maintenance therapy.[5,6]

Mithramycin

A subchemotherapeutic dose of mithramycin is an alternative approach to the urgent correction of hypercalcaemia. Mithramycin is a potent osteoclast inhibitor and lowers the plasma calcium concentration in 6–48 h. It is effective in > 80% of patients.

- give 25 mcg/kg (approximately 1.5 mg) by IV infusion over 2 h or by slow IV injection
- repeat after 48 h, up to 150 mcg/kg (< 10 mg) during the first week
- if renal function impaired, reduce dose to 15 mcg/kg (approximately 1 mg) for a single dose; 100 mcg/kg (< 7 mg) during the first week
- do not use if bone marrow suppression or unexplained bleeding tendency.

Table 6.2 Bisphosphonates and the treatment of hypercalcaemia[7]

Characteristic	Bisphosphonates		
	Pamidronate	Clodronate	Etidronate
Initial IV dose	30–60 mg	(a) 1500 mg (b) 300–600 mg daily for 5 days	7.5 mg/kg daily for 3 days
Onset of effect	< 3 days	< 2 days	< 2 days
Maximum effect	5–7 days	3–5 days	4–6 days
Duration of effect	3 weeks ±	(a) 10 days ± (b) 15 days ±	10–12 days
Reduces hypercalcaemia	< 100%	< 100%	< 100%
Restores normocalcaemia	70–90%	40–80%	15–40%
Mechanism of action inhibits osteoclasts stimulates osteoblasts	+ +	+ –	+ –
Initial PO treatment	Effective but gastro-intestinal intolerance common	Effective	Ineffective
Maintenance	IV infusion every 3–4 weeks	PO tablets generally prevent relapse	PO tablets delay relapse < 4 weeks

Calcitonin

Salmon calcitonin has a rapid calcium lowering effect which is evident within 2 h. It inhibits both osteoclast activity and renal tubular re-absorption of calcium. It is generally given SC or IM but PR is also effective. The maximum effect is seen with 100 IU/day; the effect lasts 2–3 days. More calcitonin is less effective because of 'down regulation' of calcitonin receptors in osteo-clasts. Relapse is delayed to 6–9 days by the concurrent use of a corticosteroid.[8] Long term, however, the combination of calcitonin and corticosteroids is not as efficacious as bisphosphonates or mithramycin. The main use of calcitonin is to obtain a rapid early effect when it is used together with a bisphosphonate.

Phosphate

IV neutral phosphate is effective and has a rapid onset of action. The calcium concentration begins to fall within minutes of starting an infusion; insoluble calcium-phosphate complexes are deposited in bone and soft tissues. Phosphate also inhibits osteoclast activity.

- invariably effective
- effect lasts 2–3 days
- may cause hypotension and acute renal failure, particularly if pre-existing hyperphosphataemia and renal dysfunction.

Oral inorganic phosphate 2–3 g/day restores normocalcaemia in about one third of cases. In the UK, a convenient 500 mg effervescent tablet is available. Nausea and diarrhoea are the main adverse effects and limit the dose which is tolerated. Beware of cumulation in renal failure; do not use if plasma phosphate > 5 mg/dl.

Corticosteroids

Corticosteroids are no longer recommended for hypercalcaemia associated with malignancy because of a generally poor response.[8] They are beneficial, however, when used as an adjunct to SC calcitonin.[9]

If alternative more effective treatments are not available, the use of prednisolone 60 mg o.d. or dexamethasone 8 mg o.d. should be considered in patients with breast and renal cancer or with myeloma and lymphoma.[10] Smaller doses are likely to be ineffective.

Octreotide

Octreotide is a somatostatin analogue. It has been used successfully in the treatment of hypercalcaemia associated with neuro-endocrine tumours resistant to other measures.[11]

Syndrome of inappropriate antidiuresis (SIAD)

Incidence

All malignant disease 2%.

Small cell lung cancer 10%.[12]

Causes

In cancer-related SIAD there is ectopic secretion of arginine vasopressin (antidiuretic hormone) or vasopressin-like peptides by the cancer.[13,14] In small cell lung cancer, an elevated arginine vasopressin can be detected in about 40% of patients, but the incidence of SIAD is less than 10%. There are many other causes of SIAD (Table 6.3), including antidepressants (Box 6.B). Most cases associated with SSRIs involve elderly people, particularly women.[15,16]

Table 6.3 Causes of SIAD

Caused by cancer	*Concurrent causes*
Small cell lung	Meningitis
Carcinoid	Encephalitis
Pancreas	Subarachnoid haemorrhage
Prostate	Cerebral thrombosis
Lymphoma	Pneumonia
Acute myeloid leukaemia	Tuberculosis
	Lung abscess
Caused by treatment	Schizophrenia
	Psychosis
After neurosurgery	Recreational drugs
Chemotherapy	ethanol
cyclophosphamide	nicotine
vincristine	
Drugs	
phenothiazines	
lorazepam	
barbiturates	
tricyclic antidepressants	
SSRIs	
carbamazepine	
morphine	

Box 6.B   Antidepressants and hyponatraemia (Advice of Committee on Safety of Medicines UK)

Hyponatraemia (generally in the elderly and possibly caused by SIAD) has been associated with all types of antidepressants and should be considered in all patients who develop drowsiness, confusion or convulsions while taking an antidepressant.

Clinical features

Clinical features depend on both the level and the rate of decline of plasma sodium concentration. Given time, brain cells can compensate against cerebral oedema by secreting potassium and other solutes; asymptomatic hyponatraemia therefore indicates chronic rather than acute SIAD.

Plasma sodium 110–120 mmol(mEq)/l

* anorexia

* nausea

* vomiting

* lassitude

* confusion

* oedema.

Plasma sodium < 110 mmol(mEq)/l

* multifocal myoclonus

* drowsiness

* convulsions

* coma.

Diagnosis

To be certain of the diagnosis of SIAD the following criteria should be met[17]

* hyponatraemia (< 135 mmol(mEq)/l)

* low plasma osmolality (< 270 mosmol/l)

- raised urine osmolality (> 100 mosmol/l)
- urine sodium concentration:
  always > 20 mmol(mEq)/l
  often > 50 mmol(mEq)/l
- normal plasma volume.

In practice, a plasma sodium concentration of ≤ 120 mmol(mEq)/l is sufficient to make a clinical diagnosis of SIAD in the absence of

- severe vomiting
- diuretic therapy
- hypo-adrenalism
- hypothyroidism
- severe renal failure.

Management

Treat the patient and not the biochemical results. For symptomatic patients, several therapeutic options exist

- demeclocycline 300 mg b.d.–q.d.s. acts by inducing a nephrogenic diabetes insipidus; treatment of choice in palliative care
- restrict fluid intake to 700–1000 ml/day or daily urine output to < 500 ml
- oral urea 30 g in 100 ml orange juice o.d. acts as an osmotic diuretic and obviates the need for fluid restriction
- IV hypertonic saline is not without risk; tetraparesis and bulbar palsy may develop after 1–2 days as a result of pontine myelinosis. Hypertonic saline is inappropriate in palliative care.

References

1 Ling PJ *et al.* (1995) Analysis of survival following treatment of tumour-induced hypercalcaemia with intravenous pamidronate (APD). *British Journal of Cancer.* **72**: 206–209.
2 Ralston SH *et al.* (1990) Cancer-associated hypercalcaemia: morbidity and mortality. *Annals of Internal Medicine.* **112**: 449–504.

3   Hortobagyi GN *et al.* (1996) Efficacy of pamidronate in reducing skeletal complications in patients with breast cancer and lytic bone metastases. *New England Journal of Medicine.* **335**: 1785–1791.

4   Vinholes J *et al.* (1996) Metabolic effects of pamidronate in patients with metastatic bone disease. *European Journal of Cancer.* **5**: 159–175.

5   Vorreuther R (1993) Bisphosphonates as an adjunct to palliative therapy of bone metastases from prostatic carcinoma. A pilot study on clodronate. *British Journal of Urology.* **72**: 792–795.

6   O'Rourke N *et al.* (1995) Double-blind, placebo-controlled, dose response trial of oral clodronate in patients with bone metastases. *Journal of Clinical Oncology.* **13**: 929–934.

7   Ralston SH (1994) Pathogenesis and management of cancer-associated hypercalcaemia. In: GW Hanks (ed) *Cancer Surveys, vol 21: Palliative Medicine: Problem areas in pain and symptom management.* Cold Spring Harbor Laboratory Press. pp 179–196.

8   Percival RC *et al.* (1984) Role of glucocorticoids in management of malignant hypercalcaemia. *British Medical Journal.* **289**: 287.

9   Ralston SH *et al.* (1985) Comparison of aminohydroxypropylidene bisphosphonate, mithramycin and corticosteroids/calcitonin in treatment of cancer-associated hypercalcaemia. *Lancet.* **ii**: 907–910.

10 Mannheimer IH (1965) Hypercalcaemia of breast cancer: management with corticosteroids. *Cancer.* **18**: 679–691.

11 Harrison M *et al.* (1990) Somatostatin analogue treatment for malignant hypercalcaemia. *British Medical Journal.* **300**: 1313–1314.

12 van Oosterhout AG *et al.* (1996) Neurologic disorders in 203 consecutive patients with small cell lung cancer. *Cancer.* **77**: 1434–1441.

13 Meinders AE (1993) Hyponatraemia: SIADH or SIAD? *Netherlands Journal of Medicine.* **43**: 1–4.

14 Sorensen JB *et al.* (1995) Syndrome of inappropriate secretion of antidiuretic hormone (SIADH) in malignant disease. *Journal of Internal Medicine.* **238**: 97–110.

15 ADRAC (Adverse Drug Reactions Advisory Committee) (1996) Selective serotonin reuptake inhibitors and SIADH. *Medical Journal of Australia.* **164**: 562.

16 Liu BA *et al.* (1996) Hyponatremia and the syndrome of inappropriate secretion of antidiuretic hormone associated with the use of selective serotonin reuptake inhibitors: a review of spontaneous reports. *Canadian Medical Association Journal.* **155**: 519–527.

17 Saito T (1996) SIADH and other hyponatremic disorders: diagnosis and therapeutic problems. *Japanese Journal of Nephrology.* **38**: 429–434.

7 Respiratory symptoms

Cough · Dyspnoea · Hiccup · Death rattle
Noisy tachypnoea in the moribund

Cough

Description

Cough is a complex respiratory reflex designed to expel particles and excess mucus from the trachea and main bronchi.

Cough is a protective mechanism; only when it is perceived as excessive does it become a symptom. Prolonged bouts of coughing are exhausting and frightening, particularly if they exacerbate dyspnoea or are associated with haemoptysis. Cough may also lead to nausea and vomiting, musculoskeletal pain and rib fracture.

Relevant physiology

Cough can be initiated by a wide range of receptors (Figure 7.1). There are three primary causes

- inhaled foreign matter
- excessive bronchial secretions
- abnormal stimulation of receptors in the airways.

An example of the third cause is cough caused by ACE inhibitors, seen in 20% of subjects in controlled trials.[1] The most likely mechanism is the inhibition of the breakdown of bradykinin, an inflammatory mediator. This is known to cause cough if inhaled. ACE inhibitors may also increase other local inflammatory mediators such as PGs and substance P.[2]

ACE inhibitor cough generally develops within 4 weeks of starting treatment and resolves within a similar period if treatment is stopped. It is often more troublesome at night. In about 25%, the cough necessitates the withdrawal of the ACE inhibitor.

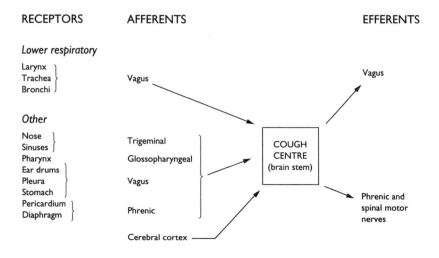

RECEPTORS   AFFERENTS   EFFERENTS

Lower respiratory

Larynx
Trachea   Vagus   Vagus
Bronchi

Other

Nose
Sinuses   Trigeminal   COUGH
Pharynx   Glossopharyngeal   CENTRE
Ear drums   (brain stem)
Pleura   Vagus
Stomach
Pericardium   Phrenic   Phrenic and
Diaphragm   spinal motor
                                                               nerves
               Cerebral cortex

Figure 7.1   The cough reflex.

Causes

Table 7.1   Causes of coughing in advanced cancer

Cardiopulmonary	*Oesophageal*
Postnasal drip	Gastro-oesophageal reflux
Smoking	
Asthma	*Aspiration*
COPD	Gastro-oesophageal reflux
Cardiac failure	Motor neurone disease
Chest infection	Multiple sclerosis
Radiation pneumonitis	Stroke
Tumour	
lung	*Medication*
mediastinum	ACE inhibitors
Vocal cord paralysis	Ipratropium
Lymphangitis carcinomatosa	Nebulized water
Effusion	
pleural	
pericardial	

Types of cough

- wet cough and patient able to cough effectively
- wet cough but patient too weak to cough effectively
- dry cough, i.e. nonproductive of sputum.

Management

Management depends on both the cause and the therapeutic goal. In the dying patient the goal is comfort. Thus, in patients who have a wet cough but are too weak to cough effectively, antitussives should be used to sedate the cough. Suction is generally not advisable; it tends to be more distressing to the patient than a pharyngeal rattle.

Explanation
Treat reversible causes (Table 7.2)

It takes 2–4 weeks to obtain significant antitussive benefit from stopping smoking. Will the patient live this long?

The newer angiotensin-II receptor antagonists, e.g. losartan, do not inhibit bradykinin breakdown and do not therefore cause cough. They can be used, if necessary, instead of an ACE inhibitor.

Nondrug measures

- advise how to cough effectively; it is impossible to cough effectively lying on your back
- postural drainage
- physiotherapy.

Drugs

There is a wide range of drugs which ease coughing (Table 7.3). Generally at Sobell House, only simple linctus and opioids are used; occasionally, a patient may need nebulized saline. The following, however, should be noted

- irritant mucolytics stimulate the production of more profuse, less viscid bronchial secretions which are easier to expectorate; *they are also gastric irritants and may cause nausea and vomiting*

Table 7.2   Reversible causes of cough

Cause	Treatment
Cigarettes	Stop smoking
Postnasal drip	Antihistamine
Respiratory infection	Antibiotic (if purulent sputum) Expectorant Physiotherapy
COPD/asthma	Bronchodilator Corticosteroid Physiotherapy
Cardiac failure	Diuretic ACE inhibitor Digoxin
ACE inhibitor	Reduce dose or stop drug Prescribe losartan instead
Oesophageal reflux	Patient should sleep semi-upright Stop or reduce dose of drug causing a reduction of lower oesophageal sphincter tone (see p.184) Metoclopramide, cisapride to increase lower oesophageal sphincter tone Proton pump inhibitor to reduce acid content and volume of gastric secretion
Aspiration of saliva	Anticholinergic to reduce saliva
Pleural effusion	Thoracentesis Pleurodesis
Malignant obstruction	Corticosteroids Radiation therapy Chemotherapy

- chemical mucolytics modify the chemical structure of sputum and thereby reduce its viscosity; best given by nebulizer
- although an opioid, pethidine is not antitussive.

Table 7.3 Drugs for cough

Mucolytics/expectorants	*Peripheral antitussives*
Saline 2–5% in nebulizer	Simple linctus
Chemical inhalations	Benzonatate (USA)
compound benzoin tincture (Friar's balsam)	Nebulized bupivacaine
carbol	
menthol and eucalyptus	*Central antitussives*
	Nonopioids
Irritant mucolytics	iso-aminile
Ammonium chloride	Opioid derivatives
Guaiphenesin	dextromethorphan
Ipecacuanha	levopropoxyphene (USA)
Potassium iodide	pholcodine
Terpin hydrate	Opioids
	codeine
Chemical mucolytics	dihydrocodeine
	hydrocodone (USA)
Acetylcysteine	morphine
Carbocysteine	methadone
	hydromorphone

Many commercial cough preparations contain suboptimal doses of an anti-tussive, a mucolytic, a sympathomimetic and an antihistamine in a demulcent (soothing) vehicle. The vehicle is probably the most important component and, like simple syrup, acts by reducing pharyngeal sensitivity.

Nebulized bupivacaine is used for refractory cough at some centres

- blocks cough receptors in the carina and bronchioles

- needs a nebulizer which gives a particle size of 2–10 Ångstrom

- use 0.5% bupivacaine 5 ml q4h

- maximum recommended dose 30 ml/24 h.

Anaesthesia of the mouth and pharynx is minimal because of the laminar flow. Some patients find the taste of bupivacaine too unpleasant.

Dyspnoea

Description

Dyspnoea is an unpleasant awareness of difficulty in breathing.

Breathlessness is what the patient reports; tachypnoea (fast breathing) and hyperpnoea (increased depth of respiration) are what the doctor measures, but neither is diagnostic of dyspnoea – which is always subjective.

Dyspnoea is more common, and often more severe, in the last few weeks before death. If dyspnoeic at rest, the patient is likely to be anxious as well.

Relevant physiology

Respiration is controlled by the respiratory centres in the brain stem (Figure 7.2). The volume of breathing is determined largely by chemical stimuli in the blood and the pattern of breathing by mechanical stimuli in the lungs, relayed in the vagus nerves. Respiratory function is modulated by various drives (Table 7.4).

Dyspnoea is usually associated with *tachypnoea*. If the resting respiratory rate is 30–35/min, activity or additional anxiety may increase this to 50–60/min.

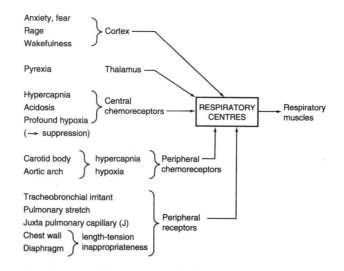

Figure 7.2 Physiology of respiration. J receptors are stimulated in both pulmonary oedema and lymphangitis carcinomatosa.

Table 7.4 Respiratory drives

Wakefulness	Lung deflation
Anxiety, fear	Acidosis
Anger, rage	Hypercapnia
Pyrexia	Hypoxia
Lung distortion	

An increased respiratory rate results in

- a relative increase in dead-space ventilation
- decreased tidal volume
- decreased alveolar ventilation.

Respiratory panic attacks

Some patients with effort dyspnoea experience respiratory panic attacks. These are often brought on by activity, e.g. going upstairs. During these attacks the patient is convinced he is going to die:

dyspnoea + lack of understanding + fear → increased anxiety → increased respiratory rate → increased dyspnoea etc.

Causes

Dyspnoea often has several concurrent causes (Table 7.5).

Evaluation

Determine the cause of any recent deterioration. Rapid changes commonly present opportunities for corrective therapy, such as pleural aspiration or antibiotics.

Management

Explanation

Respond to or anticipate the patient's questions, e.g. 'Will I choke to death?', 'Will I suffocate?', 'Will I stop breathing if I go to sleep?'

Table 7.5   Causes of dyspnoea in advanced cancer

Caused by cancer	Related to cancer and/or debility
Pleural effusion(s)	Anaemia
Obstruction of main bronchus	Atelectasis
Replacement of lung by cancer	Pulmonary embolism
Lymphangitis carcinomatosa	Pneumonia
Mediastinal obstruction	Empyema
Pericardial effusion	Cachexia-anorexia syndrome
Massive ascites	Weakness
Abdominal distension	
	Concurrent causes
Caused by treatment	COPD
Radiation-induced fibrosis	Asthma
Chemotherapy	Heart failure
bleomycin	Acidosis
doxorubicin	

Emphasize, 'Becoming breathless in itself is not dangerous', and 'Although you may feel you are suffocating when gasping for breath, you have always recovered – and you always will.'

Treat reversible causes (Table 7.6)

Nondrug measures

- a calming presence
- sight of other people
- cool draught (open window, fan)
- breathing exercises
- oxygen via nasal prongs; benefit not correlated with degree of hypoxia
- relaxation therapy
- complementary therapies, e.g.
    massage
    visualization
    acupuncture
    hypnosis.

Table 7.6 Specific treatment of dyspnoea in advanced cancer

Cause	Treatment
Respiratory infection	Antibiotic Expectorant Physiotherapy
COPD/asthma	Bronchodilators Corticosteroids Physiotherapy
Bronchial obstruction/lung collapse Mediastinal obstruction	Corticosteroids Radiotherapy LASER therapy Stent
Lymphangitis carcinomatosa	Corticosteroids
Pleural effusion	Aspiration Pleuradesis
Ascites	Diuretics (see p.218) Paracentesis
Pericardial effusion	Paracentesis Corticosteroids
Anaemia	Blood transfusion
Cardiac failure	Diuretics ACE inhibitors
Pulmonary embolism	Anticoagulants (?)

Modify way of life

- sit to wash/shave
- help with housework
- bed downstairs
- organize daily activities, i.e. eat, rest, wash, rest, dress, rest etc.

Drugs for dyspnoea

- bronchodilators may well help and should be tried; salbutamol increases voluntary muscle strength[3]

- morphine reduces respiratory drive and eases the sensation of dyspnoea:
  if on morphine for pain, increase the dose by 50%
  if not on oral morphine, 5–6 mg q4h is a good starting dose.

Nebulized morphine is not recommended; it is no better than saline.[4]

- diazepam if the patient is very anxious:
  5–10 mg stat and nocte
  in the very elderly, 2–5 mg
  reduce dose after several days if drowsy

- cannabinoids, e.g. nabilone 100 mcg q.d.s., are used at some centres in patients with severe dyspnoea in danger of developing hypercapnic respiratory failure if given opioids or benzodiazepines. With higher doses most patients complain of unacceptable sedation and some of dysphoria; hypotension and tachycardia may also be limiting factors[5]

- oxygen 4 l/min via nasal prongs if:
  dyspnoeic at rest
  acute severe dyspnoea.

Unless dyspnoeic at rest, oxygen should be discouraged except perhaps for several minutes immediately before and after physical activity. The benefit of oxygen is not dependent on correction of hypoxaemia; a trial of therapy is the only way to determine benefit, not improvement in blood gases.[6]

Respiratory panic attacks

- education about and practice in breathing control
- a calming presence
- a trial of diazepam 5–10 mg PO nocte.

Hiccup

Description

Hiccup is a pathological respiratory reflex characterized by spasm of the diaphragm, resulting in sudden inspiration and abrupt closure of the glottis with associated characteristic sound.

Causes

There are innumerable potential causes of hiccup. In advanced cancer, the following account for most cases

- gastric distension
- diaphragmatic irritation
- phrenic nerve irritation
- toxicity:
  uraemia
  infection
- CNS tumour.

Of these, gastric distension probably accounts for 95% of cases.

Acute management options

Pharyngeal stimulation (triggers a 'gating' mechanism)

Most of 'granny's remedies' for hiccup involve pharyngeal stimulation either directly or indirectly, e.g.[7]

- rapidly ingest two heaped teaspoons of granulated sugar
- rapidly ingest two glasses of liqueur
- swallow dry bread
- swallow crushed ice
- drink from the wrong side of a cup
- a cold key dropped inside the back of one's shirt or blouse
- someone shouts 'Boo!' loudly in order to produce a startle response.

Medical variations include

- forceful tongue traction sufficient to induce a gag reflex
- a nasogastric tube inserted as far as the oropharynx and jerked to-and-fro[8]
- nebulized 0.9% saline (2 ml over 5 min).[9]

Massage of the junction between hard and soft palate with a cotton bob is also an effective gating mechanism.[10]

Reduce gastric distension

- peppermint water facilitates belching by relaxing the lower oesophageal sphincter (an old-fashioned remedy)
- antiflatulent, e.g. Asilone 10 ml (a proprietary antacid containing dimeticone)
- metoclopramide 10 mg (tightens the lower oesophageal sphincter and hastens gastric emptying).

Peppermint water and metoclopramide should not be used concurrently.

Elevation of pCO_2

This inhibits processing of the hiccup reflex in the brain stem

- rebreathing from a paper bag
- breath holding.

Muscle relaxant

- baclofen 10 mg PO
- nifedipine 10 mg PO
- midazolam 2 mg IV, followed by 1–2 mg increments every 3–5 min.

Central suppression of hiccup reflex

- haloperidol 5–10 mg PO or IV if no response
- chlorpromazine 10–25 mg PO or IV if no response.

Maintenance treatment

Gastric distension

- antiflatulent, e.g. Asilone 10 ml q.d.s. *and/or*
- metoclopramide 10 mg q.d.s.

Diaphragmatic irritation or other cause

- baclofen 5–10 mg b.d.–20 mg q8h
- nifedipine 10–20 mg q8h, occasionally more[11]
- haloperidol 2–3 mg nocte
- midazolam 10–60 mg/24 h by SC infusion if all else fails.[12]

Death rattle

Description

Death rattle is a term used to describe the noise produced by the oscillatory movements of secretions in the hypopharynx, trachea or main bronchus, in association with the inspiratory and expiratory phases of respiration.

While not pathognomonic of imminent death, death rattle is generally seen only in patients who are too weak to expectorate.

Management

General

- position semiprone to encourage postural drainage
- explanation to the relatives.

Most patients dislike suctioning; it should generally be reserved for unconscious patients. Use in this circumstance is purely cosmetic, i.e. for the benefit of the relatives, other patients and staff.

Antisecretory drugs

An antisecretory drug is best started sooner rather than later because it does not affect existing pharyngeal secretions. Such drugs have less impact when the rattle is secondary to pneumonia[13] and little effect in pulmonary oedema.

Hyoscine *butylbromide* is used at Sobell House, mainly because it is cheaper, generally 20 mg stat and 20 mg/24 h by SC infusion.

Transdermal hyoscine *hydrobromide* 0.5 mg/72 h is sufficient in some patients,[14] but most need a higher dose. Many centres use hyoscine *hydrobromide* 1.2 mg/24 h and some glycopyrronium 0.6 mg/24 h by SC infusion, after an initial stat dose. Hyoscine *hydrobromide* also acts centrally (*see* p.350). Glycopyrronium is 3 times more potent than hyoscine as an antisecretory agent, and is effective in some patients who fail to respond to hyoscine.

Antisecretory drugs are effective in 50–60% of patients. However, provided time is taken to explain the cause of the rattle to the relatives and there is ongoing support, relatives' distress is relieved in > 90% of cases.[15]

Noisy tachypnoea in the moribund

Noisy tachypnoea in the moribund is distressing for the family and other patients, even though the patient is not aware. It represents a desperate last attempt by a patient's body to respond to irreversible terminal respiratory failure +/– airways obstruction. Because of the impression of patient distress, consider slowing down the respiratory rate to 10–15/min with IV diamorphine/morphine.

It may be necessary to give double or treble the previously satisfactory analgesic dose to contain this form of tachypnoea. The aim is to reduce the noise by reducing the rate and depth of respiration. If there is associated heaving of the shoulders and chest, midazolam should be given as well, e.g. 10 mg SC stat and hourly as needed.

References

1 Yeo WW *et al.* (1991) Prevalence of persistent cough during long-term enalapril treatment: controlled study versus nifedipine. *Quarterly Journal of Medicine.* **293**: 763–770.

2 Anonymous (1994) Cough caused by ACE inhibitors. *Drug and Therapeutics Bulletin.* **32**: 28.

3 Martineau L *et al.* (1992) Salbutamol, a β_2-adrenoceptor agonist, increases skeletal muscle strength in young men. *Clinical Science.* **83**: 615–621.

4 Davis C *et al.* (1996) Single dose randomized controlled trial of nebulized morphine in patients with cancer related breathlessness. *Palliative Medicine.* **10**: 64–65.

5 Ahmedzai S (1993) Palliation of respiratory symptoms. In: D Doyle, GW Hanks and N MacDonald (eds) *Oxford Textbook of Palliative Medicine.* Oxford University Press, Oxford. pp 349–378.

6 Booth S *et al.* (1996) Does oxygen help dyspnea in patients with cancer? *American Journal of Respiratory and Critical Care Medicine.* **153**: 1515–1518.

7 Lamphier TA (1977) Methods of management of persistent hiccup (singultus). *MD State Medical Journal.* **November**: 80–81.

8 Salem MR *et al.* (1967) Treatment of hiccups by pharyngeal stimulation in anesthetized and conscious subjects. *Journal of the American Medical Association.* **202**: 126–130.

9 De Ruysscher D *et al.* (1996) Treatment of intractable hiccup in a terminal cancer patient with nebulized saline. *Palliative Medicine.* **10**: 166–167.

10 Goldsmith S (1983) A treatment for hiccups. *Journal of the American Medical Association.* **249**: 1566.

11 Brigham B and Bolin T (1992) High dose nifedipine and fludrocortisone for intractable hiccups. *Medical Journal of Australia.* **157**: 70.

12 Wilcock A and Twycross R (1996) Case report: midazolam for intractable hiccup. *Journal of Pain and Symptom Management.* **12**: 59–61.

13 Bennett MI (1996) Death rattle: an audit of hyoscine (scopolamine) use and review of management. *Journal of Pain and Symptom Management.* **12**: 229–233.

14 Dawson HR (1989) The use of transdermal scopolamine in the control of death rattle. *Journal of Palliative Care.* **5** (1): 31–33.

15 Hughes A *et al.* (1997) Management of 'death rattle'. *Palliative Medicine.* **11**: 80–81.

8 Alimentary symptoms

Halitosis · Dry mouth · Stomatitis · Oral candidiasis
Abnormal taste · Failure to eat · Dehydration · Cachexia
Dysphagia · Endo-oesophageal intubation · Heartburn
Dyspepsia · Nausea and vomiting · Bowel obstruction
Constipation · Faecal impaction · Diarrhoea
Rectal discharge · Ascites

Halitosis

Definition

Halitosis means unpleasant or foul-smelling breath.

Causes

- poor dental and oral hygiene
- necrosis and sepsis in the mouth, pharynx, nose, nasal sinuses or lungs
- severe infection
- gastric stagnation associated with gastric outflow obstruction
- ingestion of substances whose volatile products are excreted by the lungs or saliva, e.g. garlic, onions, alcohol
- smoking.

Management

General measures

- clean teeth with toothbrush and paste b.d.
- consider use of dental floss or dental tape
- encourage fluid intake
- offer refreshing mouthwashes (see p.160)
- treat oral candidiasis (see p.165).

Oropharyngeal malignancy

- prescribe an appropriate antibiotic if infection present

- gargles and/or mouthwashes on waking, after meals and at bedtime:
    cider and soda water in equal parts *or*
    hydrogen peroxide 6% BP *or*
    phenol 1.4% *or*
    povidone-iodine 1%

- consider artificial saliva if the mouth is very dry (*see* p.162).

Lung sepsis

The patient generally complains of abundant foul-smelling sputum and there may be abnormal physical signs in the chest.

- send sputum for culture and prescribe an antibiotic, e.g. amoxycillin 500 mg q8h for 7 days

- if suspect necrotic cancer and anaerobic infection, prescribe metronidazole 400 mg b.d.–t.d.s. for 10 days

- if pulmonary candidiasis (rare), prescribe ketoconazole 200 mg b.d. or fluconazole 100 mg PO for 7 days.

Dry mouth

Causes

Dryness of the mouth may be caused by

- diminished secretion of saliva

- diseased buccal mucosa

- excessive evaporation of fluid from the mouth (Table 8.1).

Table 8.1 Causes of dry mouth in advanced cancer

Caused by cancer	Related to cancer and/or debility
Erosion of buccal mucosa	Anxiety
Replacement of salivary glands by cancer	Depression
	Mouth breathing
Hypercalcaemia	Dehydration
	Infection
Caused by treatment	candidiasis
	parotitis
Local radiotherapy	Fever
Local radical surgery	
Stomatitis associated with neutropenia	*Concurrent causes*
Drugs	Uncontrolled diabetes mellitus
anticholinergics (*see* p.352)	Hypothyroidism
opioids	Auto-immune disease
diuretics	Amyloid
Oxygen without humidification	Sarcoid

Management

Explanation

Encourage the patient to take frequent sips of water, preferably ice-cold, or mineral water. Mix carbonated with plain in equal parts to maintain freshness but decrease excessive gas content, or according to personal taste.

Review drug regimen

Reduce the dose of anticholinergic drugs if possible. Substitute a drug with less or no anticholinergic effects, e.g. desipramine or an SSRI instead of amitriptyline, and haloperidol instead of prochlorperazine or chlorpromazine.

Mouth care

Offer a mouthwash q2h. Effervescent mouthwash tablets (dissolve in 100 ml of water) contain peppermint oil, clove oil, spearmint, menthol, thymol and methylsalicylic acid and make a palatable and refreshing mouthwash.

Glycerine and thymol tablets are *not* recommended because glycerine produces a rebound of drying of the mouth.

Debride the tongue if furred, e.g.

- soft toothbrush and cider and soda water in equal parts *or*
- soft toothbrush and hydrogen peroxide 6% *or*
- one quarter of 1 g effervescent ascorbic acid tablet placed on the tongue.

Pineapple chunks are sometimes helpful. They contain ananase, a proteolytic enzyme, which cleans the mouth if sucked like a sweet. Fresh pineapple contains more ananase than tinned pineapple but either can be used.

A small amount (e.g. 0.5 ml) of butter, margarine or vegetable oil swished around the mouth with the tongue t.d.s. and nocte may be helpful.[1]

In moribund patients

- the mouth should be moistened with water from a water spray, dropper or sponge stick
- ice chips can be placed in the mouth every 30 min
- petroleum jelly smeared on the lips q4h will prevent cracking
- a room humidifier or air conditioning helps if the weather is dry and hot.

Stimulate salivary flow

Solids and acids in the mouth act as salivary stimulants, e.g.

- ice chips
- chewing gum
- acid drops, lemon drops, boiled sweets, strong candy
- sips of ice-cold and/or carbonated lemon drinks
- sips of 2% citric acid solution.

Pilocarpine is a parasympathomimetic agent (predominantly muscarinic) with mild β-adrenergic activity which stimulates secretion from exocrine glands, including radiation-damaged salivary glands.[2] Pilocarpine also increases the concentration of mucins in saliva; these protect the oral mucosa from trauma and dryness.

About 50% of patients with dry mouth are helped by pilocarpine. Start with 2.5–5 mg t.d.s. and increase if necessary to 10 mg t.d.s. Bowel obstruction, asthma and COPD are contra-indications to its use. The most common adverse effect is sweating; others include nausea, flushing, urinary frequency, intestinal colic and weakness.

Artificial saliva

Several proprietary artificial salivas are available in the UK, including

- pastilles containing acacia, malic acid etc. (Salivix)
- porcine gastric mucin spray and lozenges (Saliva Orthana)
- carmellose-based sprays (Glandosane, Luborant, Salivace)
- hydroxyethylcellulose-based gel (Oralbalance); contains salivary peroxidase which enhances the production of hypothiocyanite, an antibacterial ion.

Use as needed. Alternatively, methylcellulose 10 g and lemon essence 0.2 ml in 1 l of water can be used; give 1 ml every hour by dropper.

Treat oral candidiasis (see p.165)

Stomatitis

Description

Stomatitis is a general term applied to diffuse inflammatory, erosive and ulcerative conditions affecting the lining of the mouth (synonym: sore mouth).

Pathogenesis

Radiotherapy

Drugs

- cytotoxics
- corticosteroids
- antibiotics.

Infection

- candidiasis
- aphthous ulcers.

Dry mouth (see p.159)

Malnutrition

- hypovitaminosis
- anaemia
- protein deficiency.

Altered immunity

Management

Specific measures

- treat dry mouth (*see* p.160)
- modify drug regimen, i.e. stop or reduce the dose of anticholinergic drugs
- treat candidiasis (*see* p.165)
- treat aphthous ulcers; these are caused by auto-immunity and opportunistic infection (Box 8.A).

Box 8.A   Treatment of aphthous ulcers

Antibiotics and antiseptics

Chlorhexidine gluconate 0.2% mouthwash (Corsodyl); rinse the mouth with 10 ml.

Tetracycline suspension 250 mg t.d.s. for 3 days; prepared by mixing the contents of a capsule with a small quantity of water; hold in the mouth for 3 min and then spit out.

Suppression of immune response

Hydrocortisone 2.5 mg lozenges (Corlan pellets) 1 q.d.s.; place in contact with the most painful ulcer.

Triamcinolone 0.1% dental paste (Adcortyl in Orabase); apply a thin layer b.d.–q.d.s. for up to 5 days; this is difficult for patients to apply.

In HIV+ patients, thalidomide 100 mg o.d. or b.d. for 10 days is sometimes used in resistant cases of mouth ulceration. It is not a licensed drug because it causes severe congenital abnormalities (absent or shortened limbs) and irreversible peripheral neuropathy. The use of thalidomide, an immuno-modulator, is best limited to centres with the necessary expertise.

Symptomatic measures

- choline salicylate gel (Bonjela)
- benzydamine gargle (Difflam) is a NSAID with a mild local anaesthetic action which is absorbed through the skin and buccal mucosa[3]
- carbenoxolone sodium:
      Bioral gel
      Bioplex mouthwash } generally used q.d.s.
- lidocaine viscous 2% applied before meals and as needed
- cocaine hydrochloride 2% solution
- diphenhydramine hydrochloride is an antihistaminic drug with a topical analgesic effect.

Solutions of cocaine are prepared extemporaneously. 10 ml (200 mg) q4h as needed is swished around the mouth for a few minutes and then spat out. Swallowing 200 mg of cocaine would act as a powerful cerebral stimulant and could lead to agitation and hallucinations.

Diphenhydramine hydrochloride is generally given as a locally prepared compound mouthwash.[4] Proprietary solutions of diphenhydramine contain alcohol 5–14%; it is advisable to use solutions with low alcohol content.[5] The simplest preparation is diphenhydramine hydrochloride (25 mg/5 ml) and magnesium hydroxide in equal parts, up to 30 ml q2h.[6] It is spread around the mouth with the tongue and then either swallowed or spat out. Alternative formulations include

- diphenhydramine in kaopectate comprising equal parts of diphenhydramine elixir (12.5 mg/5 ml) and kaopectate; the pectin in the kaopectate helps the diphenhydramine adhere to the mucosa
- stomatitis cocktail (National Cancer Institute, USA) comprising equal parts of lidocaine viscous 2%, diphenhydramine elixir (12.5 mg/5 ml), and Maalox (a proprietary antacid). Because of the lidocaine, the mouthwash is spat out after 2 min, and not swallowed.

Oral candidiasis

This generally manifests as

* white plaques on the mucosa (thin and discrete) and/or tongue (thick and confluent) *or*
* a smooth red dry painful tongue *or*
* angular stomatitis.

Causes

Most cases are associated with

* corticosteroids
* bacterial antibiotics
* diabetes mellitus
* dry mouth.

Management

Fungal antibiotics are used to treat oral candidiasis.

Topical antibiotics

* nystatin q.d.s.–q4h:
  suspension (100 000 units/ml) 1–5 ml
  pastilles (100 000 units)
  popsicles (locally prepared) 5 ml of nystatin suspension mixed with blackcurrant or other fruit juice concentrate and frozen in an ice tray with small rounded cups.

Most patients respond to a 10 day course but some need continuous treatment. Patients must remove their dentures before each dose and clean them before re-insertion. Failure to do this leads to treatment failure.

At night dentures should be soaked in water containing nystatin 5 ml or in dilute sodium hypochlorite solution (Milton).

Systemic antibiotics

These are generally more convenient than nystatin and obviate the need for denture removal at the time of administration. Even so, it is important to remove and clean the underside of the dentures every day to remove any adherent infected debris.

- ketoconazole 200 mg tablet o.d. for 5 days; take after food to reduce gastric irritation. Most patients respond but one third relapse and need retreatment; with a course > 10 days there is a risk of liver damage

- fluconazole 150 mg capsule stat; response and relapse rates similar to ketoconazole but it is more expensive. Immunosuppressed patients may need 100–200 mg o.d. indefinitely

- miconazole 125 mg/5 ml gel q.d.s. is administered by teaspoon and the patient spreads it around the mouth with the tongue; the effect is mainly systemic; tablets are also available. It is more expensive than ketoconazole and is *not* recommended.

Ketoconazole has an inhibitory effect on cytochrome P450-mediated enzymes. This results in inhibition of adrenal steroid synthesis (corticosteroids, testosterone, oestrogens, progesterone) and of the metabolism of certain drugs. Miconazole and itraconazole have the same effect. Fluconazole has minimal effect.

As a general rule, imidazole antifungals (fluconazole, ketoconazole, itraconazole, miconazole) should not be administered concurrently with cisapride (*see* p.328). A marked rise in the plasma concentration of cisapride may occur which causes prolongation of the QT interval and a risk of ventricular tachycardia. However, the likelihood of this occurring with *fluconazole 50–100 mg o.d.* is infinitesimal.

Abnormal taste

About 50% of patients with advanced cancer experience a change in taste sensation. This is not related to primary site, other alimentary symptoms or prognosis.

There are four basic tastes

- sour (acid)
- bitter (urea)
- sweet (sucrose)
- salt.

Taste alteration may be

- a general reduction in sensitivity (hypogeusia, ageusia)
- a specific reduction or increase in sensitivity (dysgeusia), e.g. in relation to sweetness but not to other tastes.

Pathogenesis

This is largely presumptive

- decreased sensitivity of taste buds
- decreased number of taste buds
- toxic dysfunction of taste buds
- nutritional deficiencies or drugs (Table 8.2).

Hypogeusia is generally made worse by poor hygiene and oral candidiasis.

Older people generally have a reduced sense of smell. A loss of sensitivity to food odours may decrease the enjoyment of food.

Table 8.2   Taste and drugs

Drug	Effect
Phenytoin	Decreased sensitivity
Insulin	Decreased sweet and salt sensitivity after prolonged use
Lidocaine	Decreased sweet and salt sensitivity
Benzocaine	Increased sour sensitivity
5-Fluoro-uracil	Alteration in bitter and sour sensitivity
Doxorubicin	
Flurazepam	Metallic taste
Levodopa	
Lithium	Dairy products taste rancid; celery intolerable

Clinical manifestations

Vague complaints that:

'Food does not taste right'

'Everything tastes like cotton wool'.

Specific complaints that:

'I can't take sweet things anymore'

'I've given up eating meat, it tastes so bitter'

'I find I have to add spoonfuls of sugar to everything'

'I have a metallic taste in my mouth'.

Management

Mouth care

- improve mouth care and dental hygiene
- treat oral candidiasis.

Modify diet

The advice of a dietician should be obtained and an appropriate recipe book supplied

- to help overcome general poor taste:
  tart foods, e.g. pickles, lemon juice, vinegar
  eat food which leaves its own taste, e.g. fresh fruit, hard candy
- add or reduce sugar as appropriate
- reduce urea content of diet, i.e. eat white meats, eggs, dairy products
- mask bitter taste of food containing urea:
  add wine and beer to soups and sauces
  marinate chicken, fish, meat
  use more and stronger seasonings
  eat food cold or at room temperature
  drink more liquids.

Failure to eat

Whose problem is it? The patient's or family's?

It is natural for people close to death to lose interest in food, and eventually in fluids. Before a natural disinterest is accepted as the main causal factor, reversible causes should be identified and corrected (Table 8.3).

Table 8.3 Causes of poor appetite in advanced cancer

Causes	Treatment possibilities
Fear of vomiting	Anti-emetic
Unappetizing food	Choice of food by patient
Too much food offered	Small meals
Early satiety	Snacks between meals
Dehydration	Rehydrate
Constipation	Laxatives
Sore mouth	Mouth care (*see* p.162)
Pain	Analgesics
Fatigue	
Malodour	Treatment of malodour (*see* p.268)
Biochemical	
hypercalcaemia	Correction of hypercalcaemia (*see* p.134)
hyponatraemia	Correction of SIAD (*see* p.141)
uraemia	Anti-emetic
Secondary to treatment	
drugs	Modify drug regimen
radiotherapy	
chemotherapy	
Disease process	Appetite stimulant (*see* p.170)
Anxiety	Anxiolytic
Depression	Antidepressant

Management

- explanation

- listen to the family's fears

- discourage the 'he must eat or he will die' syndrome by emphasizing that a balanced diet is not necessary at this stage in the illness:
    'Just give him a little of what he fancies'
    'I shall be happy even if he just takes fluids'
    'After all, babies thrive on milk'

- understand and be prepared to offer simple psychological support to overcome the 'food as love' and 'feeding him is my job' syndromes

- a small helping looks better on a smaller plate; do not use large dinner plates

- explain to the family:
    how they can assist a fickle appetite by providing food when the patient is hungry (a microwave oven helps to achieve this)
    that the patient will be satisfied with less intake, and that this is normal

- offer specific dietary advice

- remember that eating is a social habit – people generally eat better at a table and when dressed

- treatment of malodour (see p.268)

- appetite stimulants:
    corticosteroid, e.g. prednisolone 15–30 mg o.d., methylprednisolone 32 mg o.d. or dexamethasone 2–4 mg o.d.; useful in about 50% of patients but the effect may last for only a few weeks[7,8]
    progestogen, e.g. medroxyprogesterone acetate 400 mg o.d. or megesterol 160 mg o.d.; the effect may last for months and is generally associated with weight gain.[9]

Dehydration

Terminally ill patients often lose interest in food as they physically deteriorate. Moribund patients often lose interest in hydration as well but are not distressed provided the mouth is cleaned and moistened regularly.[10,11]

On the other hand, patients who develop acute dehydration, e.g. as a result of vomiting, diarrhoea or polyuria, experience distressing thirst and generally need parenteral rehydration.[12] Some patients, however, prefer not to have an infusion even in these circumstances and generally their disinclination should be respected. Remember: the aim is comfort, not a perfect fluid balance chart with normal electrolytes (Box 8.B).

For some patients, intermittent SC infusion (hypodermoclysis) is preferable to continuous IV infusion. Either 5% glucose-saline or 0.9% saline can be infused. Amounts vary between 500 ml and 2 l/24 h, given over 3–12 h through a 25 gauge needle.[13] Fluid can be administered by this route for several months in patients with, for example, head and neck cancer.

Hyaluronidase is sometimes added to the infusate.[13] It does not, however, increase comfort or absorption.[14] In patients with delirium, improved hydration may lead to improved mentation[15] – but not invariably. Hypodermoclysis is infrequently used at Sobell House.

Box 8.B   Parenteral hydration in palliative care

Indications

Generally all the following criteria should be met

- the patient is experiencing symptoms (e.g. thirst, malaise, delirium) for which dehydration seems the most likely cause

- increased oral intake not feasible

- anticipation that parenteral hydration will relieve the symptoms (e.g. in patients with severe dysphagia, vomiting or diarrhoea)

- the patient's underlying physical condition is relatively good (e.g. some patients with head and neck cancer)

- the patient is willing to have parenteral hydration

- the patient and relatives understand that the purpose is to relieve symptoms and not to cure.

It is advisable initially to give a provisional time limit for parenteral hydration, e.g. 2–3 days, after which it will be discontinued if not helpful.

Contra-indications

- the patient requests not to have an invasive procedure

- the sum of the burdens of parenteral hydration outweigh the likely benefits

- the patient is moribund for reasons other than dehydration.

If it is not in the patient's best interests, parenteral hydration should not be introduced simply to satisfy relatives who insist that something must be done.

Cachexia

Definition

Cachexia means marked weight loss and muscle wasting. It is often associated with anorexia as the cachexia-anorexia syndrome.

Causes

Cachexia occurs in over 50% of patients with advanced cancer.[16] The incidence is highest in gastro-intestinal and lung cancers.

Cachexia is not correlated with food intake or the stage of the tumour. It may antedate the clinical diagnosis and can occur with a small primary neoplasm. Cachexia is a paraneoplastic syndrome, but is exacerbated by concurrent adverse factors (Table 8.4).

Table 8.4   Causal factors of cachexia in advanced cancer[16]

Paraneoplastic	Concurrent
Increased metabolic rate → increased energy expenditure	Anorexia → deficient food intake
	Vomiting
Abnormal host metabolism of protein carbohydrate fat hormones	Diarrhoea
	Malabsorption
	Intestinal obstruction
Nitrogen trap by the tumour	Debilitating effect of treatment surgery radiotherapy chemotherapy
Cytokine production by host cells tumour, e.g. tumour necrosis factor	Ulceration ⎫ excessive loss of Haemorrhage ⎭ body protein

Clinical features

The principal features of cachexia-anorexia syndrome are

• marked weight loss

- anorexia
- weakness
- lassitude.

Associated physical features include

- altered taste sensation
- loose dentures causing pain and difficulty with eating
- pallor (anaemia)
- oedema (hypo-albuminaemia)
- pressure sores.

Psychosocial ramifications extend to

- ill-fitting clothes which increase the sense of loss and displacement
- altered appearance which engenders fear and isolation
- difficulties in social and family relationships.

Management

Because of the increased metabolic rate, aggressive dietary supplementation via a nasogastric tube or IV hyperalimentation is of little value in reversing cachexia in advanced cancer. Even so, dietary advice is important, particularly if there are associated changes in taste sensation (*see* p.166). A trial of therapy with corticosteroid, followed possibly by a progestogen is worthwhile in some patients (*see* p.170). The use of the latter, however, is often restricted by cost.

Efforts should also be directed towards ameliorating the social consequences and physical complications

- denture relining done at the bedside will last about 3 months; it restores chewing abilities and improves facial appearance
- if it can be afforded, a new set of clothes pays handsome dividends in enhanced self-esteem.

An old photo from before the weight loss will help the new caregivers recognize the essential humanness of the emaciated individual. Equally, new photos taken of the patient with the family and friends will help to legitimize the value of this 'different' person by emphasizing that he still occupies a place in the world.

The patient and family need education about the new bony prominences and the importance of skin care (see p.269). Routine weighing of the patient should be avoided.

Supply items designed to enhance personal independence in the face of weakness, e.g. wheelchair, ramps, raised toilet seat, commode, hospital bed, walking frame, mat for the bath.

Dysphagia

Definition

Dysphagia means difficulty in swallowing.

Dysphagia is the presenting symptom in most pharyngeal and oesophageal cancers. At some stage, dysphagia occurs in almost all patients with head and neck cancer. It is a feature of other cancers which spread to the mediastinum, neck, or base of skull, e.g. lung cancer and lymphoma. Nonobstructive dysphagia associated with extreme weakness and/or cachexia is also common.

Relevant physiology

Swallowing is a complex phenomenon, involving the brain stem, five cranial nerves, and 34 skeletal muscles. It comprises four distinct phases; two voluntary and two reflexive[17]

- oral preparatory phase – food is mixed with saliva and chewed to reduce particle size

- oral swallowing phase – the lips are closed to prevent leakage and the anterior tongue retracts and elevates in a wave which pushes the bolus into the oropharynx

- pharyngeal phase – this is triggered by the bolus reaching the posterior tongue. The larynx closes, breathing stops, and a peristaltic wave moves the bolus into the oesophagus in less than 1 second. These complex actions are necessary to protect the airway because the pharynx is a shared passage for air and food

- oesophageal phase – reflux peristalsis carries the bolus into the stomach.

Causes

There are many causes of dysphagia in advanced cancer (Table 8.5). Two basic processes are involved

- mechanical obstruction
- neuromuscular defects.

Evaluation

- distinguish from painful swallowing (odynophagia)
- obstructing lesions cause dysphagia for solids initially with later progression to liquids
- neuromuscular disorders cause dysphagia for both solids and liquids about the same time.

Patients can almost invariably localize the anatomical site of the problem.[17] The patient's description together with personal observation of the patient provides additional information (Table 8.6).

Management

Explanation

Explanation and agreement between patient, family and staff about feeding goals and treatment plans.

Dietary advice

- recommend suitable soft food cookbooks
- use of liquidizer/blenderizer
- add cream to soup (high caloric content)
- eat cold sour cream by the spoonful
- offer general advice about managing mealtimes (Box 8.C).

Table 8.5 Causes of dysphagia in advanced cancer

Caused by cancer

Mass lesion in mouth, pharynx or oesophagus
Linear infiltration of pharyngo-oesophageal wall
→ damage to nerve plexus
External compression (mediastinal mass)
Perineural tumour spread (vagus and sympathetic)
Tumour spread across base of skull
→ cranial nerve palsies
Metastases in base of skull
→ cranial nerve palsies
Leptomeningeal infiltration
→ cranial nerve palsies
Cerebral metastatic disease
→ bulbar palsy
Paraneoplastic

Related to cancer and/or debility

Dry mouth
Pharyngo-oesophageal candidiasis
Pharyngeal bacterial infection
Anxiety → oesophageal spasm
Drowsiness and disinterest
Extreme weakness (patient moribund)
Hypercalcaemia (rare)

Caused by treatment

Surgery
lingual
buccal
Postradiation fibrosis
difficulty in opening mouth and moving tongue
prolonged oesophageal transit
oesophageal stricture
Upward displacement of endo-oesophageal tube
Drugs (dystonic reaction)
neuroleptics
metoclopramide

Concurrent causes

Reflux oesophagitis
Benign stricture
Iron deficiency

Table 8.6 Evaluation of dysphagia[18]

Information provided	Possible interpretation
Leakage from mouth, drooling	Poor lip closure, reduced lip sensation, abnormal tongue movement or reduced/absent swallowing reflex
Bites cheeks or tongue	Reduced lip or tongue sensation
Frequent nasal regurgitation	Palatal dysfunction
Food collecting	
in mouth	Poor lip, buccal or tongue control
in vallecula/pyriform fossae	Reduced/absent swallowing reflex
Patient washes food down with a drink or pushes food in with finger	Reduced tongue control
Patient tilts head down during swallowing	Delayed swallowing reflex or poor laryngeal closure
Difficulty with solids	
in triggering swallowing	Poor tongue control
food sticks	Obstruction
Lack of awareness where food is during swallowing	Sensory loss
Difficulty with liquids	Poor tongue control, reduced/absent swallowing reflex, muscular inco-ordination, soft palate, paralysis or fixation, severe obstruction
Coughing, choking	Aspiration due to
before swallowing	poor tongue control or delayed or absent swallowing reflex
during swallowing	reduced airway protection
after swallowing	reduced pharyngeal emptying, reduced laryngeal elevation, cricopharyngeus dysfunction, pharyngeal or oesophageal obstruction or tracheo-oesophageal fistula
Voice changes	
inability to say 'pa'	Poor lip closure
inability to say 'ka'	Poor movement of posterior tongue
'gargle' type voice	Aspiration
'hot potato' voice	Vallecular tumours
'breathy' voice/hoarseness	Recurrent laryngeal nerve palsy

Box 8.C   Helpful hints to aid feeding in patients with dysphagia (adapted from Speech and Language Therapy, Frenchay Hospital, Bristol, UK)

Posture

Make sure that you are sitting comfortably, head upright.

Relax

Ensure you are in a calm frame of mind before eating and drinking.

Do not talk

Be quiet before and while you eat and drink.

Yawn

Before the meal, if your throat feels tight, try to yawn to ease the constriction.

Feeding routine

Small amount → close lips → chew → pause → purposeful swallow → pause.

Texture

Try to avoid mixing fluids and solids.

Take time

Do not hurry. Always stop eating if you feel tired. Have small regular meals, not one large one.

After the meal

Drink small amount of water to rinse your mouth out, also cough to make sure throat is clear.

Sit

Remain sitting for at least half an hour after eating or drinking.

Maintenance of lumen

- trial of corticosteroids[19]

- intermittent bouginage with blunt-tipped bougie (rarely used in UK)

- endoscopic dilation; benefits > 50% of patients but often for only 1–2 weeks

- radiotherapy (external beam or brachytherapy); benefits > 50% for a median of 4 months

- LASER treatment; benefit may last as long as brachytherapy if a retrograde approach is used[20]

- intubation (*see* p.179).

Endoscopic LASER therapy produces better relief of dysphagia than intubation.[21,22] Several treatments are generally required – more so with prograde resections. In about one quarter of the patients, restoration of the lumen does not result in an adequate oral intake.[20] Alcohol injection of the malignant obstructions produces similar results to LASER therapy and is an alternative when LASER therapy is not available.[23,24]

Maintenance of nutritional intake

- endo-oesophageal intubation (*see below*)
- Clinifeed enteric tube; transnasal placement by a doctor on the ward is possible if the oesophageal lumen > 1 cm
- feeding gastrostomy.[25]

A Clinifeed enteric tube or a feeding gastrostomy is generally contra-indicated in advanced cancer. The question arises more in patients with neurological disorders, e.g. poststroke and motor neurone disease (Figure 8.1).

Much depends on the speed of deterioration and the opinion of the patient and family, as well as those of the carers. In cases of doubt, it is better to delay several days, or even weeks, before taking the decision to go ahead. It is easier not to start a treatment than to stop it a short time later. Guidelines on artificial nutrition in terminally ill patients are available.[26,27]

Reduction of saliva

If total obstruction produces sialorrhoea and drooling, reduce salivary flow by

- prescribing an antisecretory (anticholinergic) drug:
  propantheline
  tricyclic antidepressant
  phenothiazine
  belladonna alkaloid
- irradiating the salivary glands with 4–10 Gy.

Endo-oesophageal intubation

An indwelling flexible endo-oesophageal tube (e.g. Celestin) or an expandable stent[28,29] can be used to maintain a passage for fluid and food through a narrowed portion of the oesophagus or gastro-oesophageal junction. Expandable stents are 20–30 times more expensive and functional superiority is unproven.

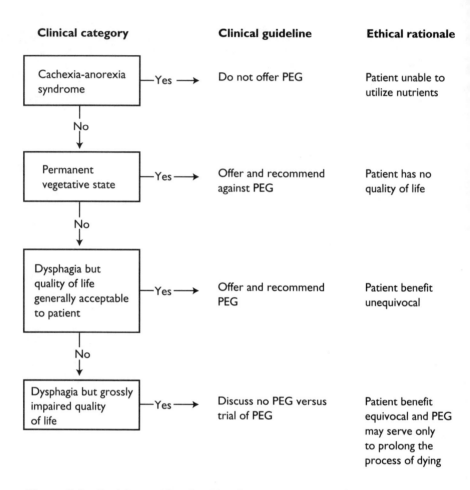

Figure 8.1   Decision-making algorithm for percutaneous endoscopic gastrostomy (PEG) tube placement. Modified from Rabenek *et al.* 1997.[30]

The upper end of the tube is broader in diameter and this both impedes downward displacement and serves as a funnel for ingested matter. The tube is introduced by a surgeon through an upper abdominal incision or via a fibre-optic gastroscope. Radiotherapy does not affect the tube.

Indications for use

- marked dysphagia for semisolids including liquidized/blenderized foods
- patient relatively independent and active.

An endo-oesophageal tube is *contra-indicated* in moribund patients.

Postoperative management

- elevate on 2 or 3 pillows to prevent reflux of gastric contents
- begin with fluid diet and change after 1–2 days to a semisolid one
- confirm position of the tube with a Gastrografin swallow 3–4 days after the operation
- introduce solids after 5–7 days; the patient must chew foods twice as long as normal (Box 8.D)
- avoid the following foods completely:
  fish – bony or without sauce
  hard boiled eggs
  oranges and other pithy fruit
- sips of a carbonated drink are taken frequently during and after every meal; less so in patients with a small stomach capacity.

The tube rarely gets blocked if advice is carefully followed (Box 8.E).

Heartburn

Definition

Heartburn is a burning retrosternal discomfort which is generally caused by the reflux of acidic gastric contents into the oesophagus.

Associated symptoms

- regurgitation
- painful swallowing
- transient distal dysphagia for solid foods only
- water brash (episodic hypersalivation)[31]
- intermittent cough or wheezing secondary to aspiration of stomach contents
- weakness caused by anaemia secondary to bleeding from oesophageal ulceration.

Box 8.D   Dietary recommendations for patients with an endo-oesophageal tube

Protein rich food

Eat	Avoid
Tender meat in gravy	Tough or dry meats
Flaked fish in sauce	Any fish with bones or without sauce
Grated cheese/cheese in sauce	Lumps of hard cheese
Soft cheese – cottage/cream	Fried or hard boiled eggs
Soft boiled and scrambled eggs	
Milk – full cream, evaporated/ condensed	

Fruit and vegetables

Include	Exclude
Fruit juices	Dried fruit – raisins, sultanas etc.
Peeled soft or stewed fruits – no pips	Nuts
Puréed tinned fruit	Raw vegetables or salads, e.g. lettuce, tomato
Yoghurts/mousses	Stringy vegetables, e.g. beans, sweetcorn, peas, cauliflower stalks, cabbage stalks
Soft well cooked mashed vegetables	Fibrous or pithy fruits, e.g. grapefruit, orange, pineapple, grapes
	Fruit skins/pips, e.g. damson jam, peach, pear or apple skin

Starches – bread, potato, cereals

Eat	Avoid
Potato – mashed with butter	Chips or roast potatoes
Boiled white rice or spaghetti	Potato crisps/snacks
Tinned spaghetti, macaroni, milk puddings	Wholegrain rice
Day old wholemeal bread with plenty of butter/margarine	Granary bread
Soft crumbly biscuits, e.g. digestive, shortbread, chocolate coated biscuits	French sticks, new white bread or bread crusts
Semisolid smooth breakfast cereals, e.g. porridge, Ready Brek, All Bran, Weetabix	Hard flaky biscuits, e.g. water biscuits
	Doughy cakes and fruit cake
	Puff pastry and Danish pastry
	Muesli, nutty cereals, Shredded Wheat

Box 8.E   General dietary advice to patients with an endo-oesophageal tube

---

A plastic tube has been put into your food pipe to help you eat and drink more easily.

Because this has an internal opening about the size of your index finger, you need to be careful about what you swallow – hard or lumpy food may block the tube.

Never take tablets unless crushed or dissolved.

Take small mouthfuls of food and chew well.

Always sip a fizzy/carbonated drink with your meal.

Eat 'little and often', e.g. 6 snacks rather than 2–3 big meals.

Food should never be eaten dry; lubricate with butter, margarine, milk, ice cream, gravy, sauce etc.

Don't use baby foods; they are designed for a baby and are low in protein and calories.

Drink more nourishing fluid and less tea, coffee, squash, water.

Continue to drink alcohol in moderation; preferably adding a fizzy/carbonated mixer to your favourite tipple and sip it with your meals, e.g. gin and tonic, beer shandy, Bucks fizz.

If your tube becomes blocked, try
- sipping a fizzy drink
- jumping
- standing up
- sipping another drink.

If this doesn't work, contact your doctor for further advice and help.

Although a blocked tube is distressing, it is not a serious medical problem.

Pathogenesis of heartburn

The distal 5 cm of the oesophagus is a high pressure zone (normally 10–12 mm Hg) which prevents reflux. This lower oesophageal sphincter relaxes with swallowing and its tone increases when the stomach is filled. Reflux occurs when the lower oesophageal sphincter becomes dysfunctional (Table 8.7).

Many drugs have an adverse effect on lower oesophageal sphincter tone (Table 8.7). The onset of heartburn within 1–2 days of commencing a new drug should alert the doctor to this possibility. The use of morphine and other opioids can cause reflux secondary to delayed gastric emptying.

Table 8.7   Factors which decrease the competence of the lower oesophageal sphincter

Dietary	*Drugs*
Alcohol	Nicotine
Chocolate	Anticholinergics
Fat	Benzodiazepines
Carminatives	Calcium-channel blockers
mint	Nitrates and nitrites
anise	Oestrogens
dill	Pethidine/meperidine
Carbonated beverages	Theophylline
Aerophagic habits	
chewing gum	*Mechanical*
sucking hard candy	
Very big meals	Constricting abdominal garments
	Obesity
	Ascites
	Lying flat

Management

Explanation

- modify diet (Table 8.7)
- stop smoking.

Nondrug measures

- avoid constricting garments and lying flat after eating
- elevate the head of the bed by 10 cm
- paracentesis if marked ascites present
- weight reduction if obese (generally not applicable in advanced cancer).

Drug measures

- stop or reduce the dose of causal drugs if possible
- change to a drug with less anticholinergic properties, e.g. substitute an SSRI for a tricyclic antidepressant
- prescribe a prokinetic to increase lower oesophageal pressure, e.g. metoclopramide or cisapride

- reduce stomach acid by prescribing an antacid (*see* p.321), an H_2-receptor antagonist or a proton pump inhibitor.

Occasional mild heartburn responds to antacids. For severe heartburn, both a proton pump inhibitor and a prokinetic should be prescribed.

Dyspepsia

Description

Dyspepsia is postprandial discomfort or pain centred in the upper abdomen (synonym: indigestion). Dyspepsia encompasses a range of symptoms (Table 8.8). These vary in intensity and are not all present in every patient or in every episode.

Table 8.8 Symptoms of dyspepsia[32]

Symptom	Comment
Epigastric pain	Mainly postprandial.
Epigastric discomfort	A negative feeling which does not reach the level of pain and which can include any of the symptoms below.
Early satiety	A feeling that the stomach is overfull soon after starting to eat so that the meal cannot be finished.
Postprandial fullness	An unpleasant sensation of persistence of food in the stomach.
Epigastric bloating	Sensation of visceral distension in the upper abdomen; this is not the same as visible abdominal distension.
Belching	
Heartburn	
Hiccup	
Nausea	
Retching	
Vomiting	

Pathogenesis

There are many cause of dyspepsia (Table 8.9). From a therapeutic perspective, dyspepsia can be divided into four categories

- small stomach capacity

- gassy

- acid

- dysmotility.

Table 8.9   Causes of dyspepsia in advanced cancer

Caused by cancer	*Related to cancer and/or debility*
Small stomach capacity	Oesophageal candidiasis
large unresected stomach cancer	Minimal food and fluid intake
linitis plastica	Anxiety → aerophagia
massive ascites	
Gastroparesis (paraneoplastic	*Concurrent causes*
visceral neuropathy)	
	Organic dyspepsia
Caused by treatment	peptic ulcer
	reflux oesophagitis
Postsurgical	cholelithiasis
postgastrectomy	renal failure
reflux oesophagitis	Non-ulcer dyspepsia
Radiotherapy	dysmotility-like
lumbar spine	aerophagia
epigastrium	
Drugs	
physical irritant (→ gastritis), e.g.	
iron	
metronidazole	
tranexamic acid	
acid stimulant (→ gastritis), e.g.	
NSAIDs	
corticosteroids	
delayed gastric emptying	
anticholinergics	
opioids	
cisplatin	

Functional dyspepsia (i.e. dyspepsia without apparent organic cause) is generally caused by dysmotility. It is seen in about 25% of the normal population and is therefore common in patients with cancer.

Most cases of squashed stomach syndrome[33] and cancer-associated dyspepsia syndrome[34] are probably examples of functional dysmotility dyspepsia exacerbated by

- opioid-induced delayed gastric emptying
- gross hepatomegaly
- gross ascites.

Some cancer patients complain of marked early satiety and/or other dyspeptic symptoms without any obvious predisposing cause.[35] This probably relates to paraneoplastic visceral autonomic neuropathy.[36] There is often associated evidence of impaired autonomic control of the cardiovascular system manifesting, for example, as postural hypotension without a compensatory tachycardia.[37]

Another cause of gastric distension is swallowed air. Licking one's lips initiates a swallowing reflex which sucks air into the stomach. A similar association is seen with sniffing, a common concomitant of acute coryza or nasal catarrh. Anxiety and smoking both increase gastric gas because the associated dry lips result in licking. Up to 15% of laryngectomees give up any attempt at oesophageal speech because of the large volumes of air which are swallowed, preferring silence to abdominal distension and pain.[38]

Evaluation

It is important to differentiate between the four types of dyspepsia because the treatment differs. Careful history taking generally indicates which type is predominant. Patients with dysmotility dyspepsia often have symptoms or a history of irritable bowel syndrome.

Management

Small stomach capacity

If dyspepsia is associated with a small stomach capacity, patients should be advised to separate their main fluid from their main solid intake, and to eat 'small and often', i.e. take 5–6 small meals/snacks during the day rather than 2–3 big meals.

Patients with a small stomach capacity may benefit from an antiflatulent after meals – to help clear space in a relatively overfull stomach.

Gassy dyspepsia

Prescribe an antiflatulent, e.g. activated dimeticone. This is available on its own but may conveniently be given in the form of Asilone, a proprietary antacid (*see* p.322). Depending on a patient's individual needs, this can be given as needed, q.d.s., or both.

Acid dyspepsia

Prescribe an antacid, H_2-receptor antagonist (e.g. cimetidine, ranitidine) or a proton pump inhibitor (e.g. lansoprazole, omeprazole).

In patients taking a NSAID, misoprostol (a PG analogue) should be used for dyspepsia, 200 mcg q.d.s. or 400 mcg b.d. If used prophylactically to prevent NSAID gastropathy in patients with a history of peptic ulceration, 200 mcg b.d. is generally adequate.

Dysmotility dyspepsia

This is not helped by gastric acid reduction. Treatment is with a prokinetic drug, i.e. metoclopramide, domperidone, cisapride (*see* p.326). These normalize disordered gastric motility.

Nausea and vomiting

Description

Nausea is an unpleasant feeling of the need to vomit, often accompanied by autonomic symptoms, i.e. pallor, cold sweat, salivation, tachycardia and diarrhoea.

Retching is rhythmic, laboured, spasmodic movements of the diaphragm and abdominal muscles, generally occurring in the presence of nausea and often culminating in vomiting.

Vomiting is the forceful expulsion of gastric contents through the mouth.

Pathogenesis

Vomiting is a complex reflex process involving co-ordinated activities of the gastro-intestinal tract, diaphragm and abdominal muscles. Nausea is an expression of autonomic stimulation; retching and vomiting are mediated via somatic nerves. Atony of the stomach, lower oesophageal sphincter and pylorus is associated with retroperistalsis. The expulsive effort of vomiting is produced by the primary and accessory muscles of respiration, notably the abdominal muscles. The emetic pattern generator (vomiting centre) co-ordinates the process, receiving and integrating input from several sources (Figure 8.2).

Relevant anatomy

The area postrema is in the floor of the 4th ventricle in the brain stem (Figure 8.3). It includes a functional entity called the chemoreceptor trigger zone. Because the area postrema lies outside the blood-brain barrier it is 'bathed' in the systemic circulation. Dopamine receptors in the area postrema are stimulated by high concentrations of emetogenic substances such as calcium ions, urea, morphine and digoxin. The area postrema also receives input from the vestibular apparatus and the vagus.

The nucleus tractus solitarius is the main central connection of the vagus and lies partly in the deeper layers of the area postrema (Figure 8.3). It contains the greatest concentration of $5HT_3$-receptors in the brain stem. The emetic pattern generator is close to the area postrema but lies fully within the blood-brain barrier. It comprises a collection of motor nuclei, including the nucleus ambiguus, ventral and dorsal respiratory groups, and the dorsal motor nucleus of the vagus.

Evaluation

- distinguish between vomiting, expectoration and regurgitation
- check fundi for papilloedema, although its absence does not exclude raised intracranial pressure
- examine the abdomen
- do a rectal examination if faecal impaction is a possibility
- consider checking:
    plasma creatinine
    plasma calcium and albumin
    plasma carbamazepine
    plasma digoxin
- review drug regimen.

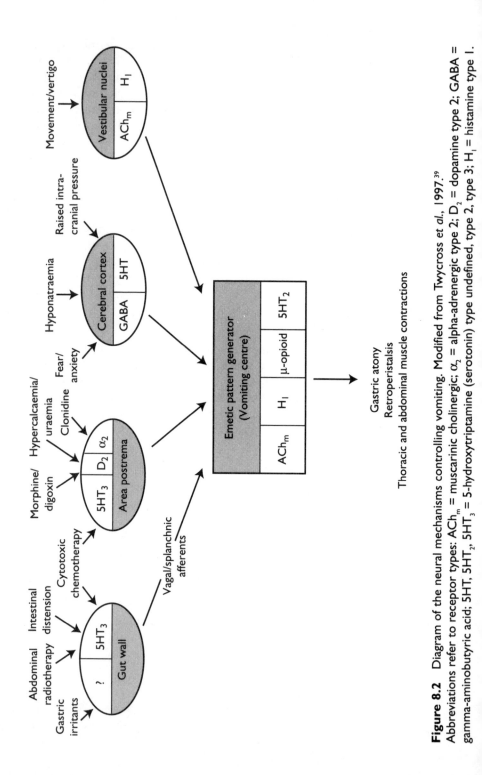

Figure 8.2 Diagram of the neural mechanisms controlling vomiting. Modified from Twycross et al., 1997.[39] Abbreviations refer to receptor types: ACh_m = muscarinic cholinergic; α_2 = alpha-adrenergic type 2; D_2 = dopamine type 2; GABA = gamma-aminobutyric acid; 5HT, $5HT_2$, $5HT_3$ = 5-hydroxytryptamine (serotonin) type undefined, type 2, type 3; H_l = histamine type l.

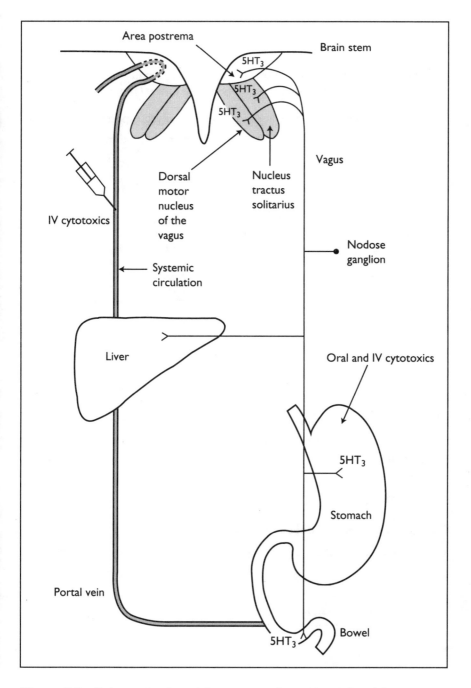

Figure 8.3 Pathways implicated in nausea and vomiting induced by cytotoxic drugs and the sites of action of 5HT$_3$-receptor antagonists. Modified from Barnes and Barnes, 1991.[40]

Causes

It is important to identify the most likely cause(s) of nausea and vomiting in each patient because treatment depends on the cause (Table 8.10).

Table 8.10   Causes of nausea and vomiting in advanced cancer

Caused by cancer	*Caused by treatment*
Gastroparesis (paraneoplastic visceral neuropathy)	Radiotherapy
	Chemotherapy
Blood in stomach	Drugs
Bowel obstruction	antibiotics
partial	aspirin
complete	carbamazepine
Constipation	corticosteroids
Hepatomegaly	digoxin
Gross ascites	iron
Raised intracranial pressure	mucolytics/expectorants
Cough	NSAIDs
Pain	oestrogens
Anxiety	opioids
Cancer toxicity	theophylline
Hypercalcaemia	
Hyponatraemia	*Concurrent causes*
Renal failure	
	Functional dyspepsia
Related to cancer and/or debility	Peptic ulcer
	Alcohol gastritis
Cough	Renal failure
Infection	

Management

Correct reversible causes

- cough → antitussive

- gastritis → reduction of gastric acid:
    antacid
    H_2-receptor antagonist
    proton pump inhibitor

- consider stopping gastric irritant drugs:
    antibiotic
    corticosteroid
    irritant mucolytic
    NSAID

- constipation → laxative
- raised intracranial pressure → corticosteroid
- hypercalcaemia → IV saline + bisphosphonate (*see* p.136).

Nondrug measures

- a calm, re-assuring environment away from the sight and smell of food
- small snacks, e.g. a few mouthfuls, and not big meals
- avoid exposure to foods which precipitate nausea; this may mean transferring the patient to a single room
- if the patient is the household cook, someone else may need to take on this role.

Drugs

Anti-emetics must be used logically and methodically (Figure 8.4). On the basis of putative sites of action (Table 8.11), it is possible to derive anti-emetic drugs of choice for different situations (Box 8.F and Table 8.12).

The initial choice generally lies between 3 drugs – metoclopramide, haloperidol and cyclizine. Second-line drugs need to be added or substituted in some patients, e.g. hyoscine butylbromide and dexamethasone. For a few, levomepromazine +/– dexamethasone will be necessary. Occasionally, a trial of a $5HT_3$ antagonist will be appropriate. This is an expensive option; if the $5HT_3$ antagonist is not clearly effective within 3 days, it should be discontinued.

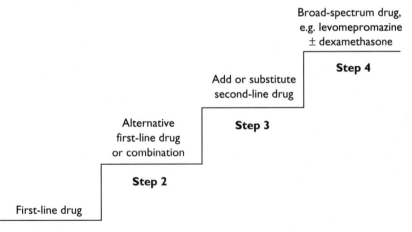

Figure 8.4   The 4-step anti-emetic ladder. To be used only after careful evaluation and with imagination (*see* Box 8.F). 'Narrow-spectrum' and 'broad-spectrum' refer to receptor site affinities (*see* Tables 8.11 and 8.12).

Table 8.11 Anti-emetic classification

Putative site of action	Class	Example
Central nervous system		
Emetic pattern generator (vomiting centre)	Anticholinergic	Hyoscine hydrobromide
	Antihistaminic anticholinergic[a]	Cyclizine, dimenhydrinate, phenothiazines
	$5HT_2$ antagonist	Levomepromazine[b]
Area postrema (chemoreceptor trigger zone)	Dopamine (D_2) antagonist	Haloperidol, phenothiazines, metoclopramide, domperidone
	$5HT_3$ antagonist	Granisetron, ondansetron, tropisetron
Cerebral cortex	Benzodiazepine	Lorazepam
	Cannabinoid	Nabilone
	Corticosteroid[c]	Dexamethasone
Gastro-intestinal tract		
Prokinetic	$5HT_4$ agonist	Metoclopramide, cisapride
	Dopamine (D_2) antagonist	Metoclopramide, domperidone
Antisecretory	Anticholinergic	Hyoscine butylbromide, glycopyrronium
	Somatostatin analogue	Octreotide, vapreotide
Vagal $5HT_3$-receptor blockade	$5HT_3$ antagonist	Granisetron, ondansetron, tropisetron
Anti-inflammatory effect	Corticosteroid[c]	Dexamethasone

a   the antihistamines and phenothiazines both have H_1 antagonist and anticholinergic properties to a variable degree

b   levomepromazine is a phenothiazine with $5HT_2$ antagonist properties; this makes it a potent broad-spectrum anti-emetic; its main disadvantages are sedation and postural hypotension

c   corticosteroids possibly act by reducing the permeability of the area postrema and of the blood-brain barrier to emetogenic substances and by reducing the neuronal content of gamma-aminobutyric acid (GABA) – an inhibitory amine – in the brain stem; corticosteroids also reduce leu-enkephalin release in both the brain stem and the gastro-intestinal tract.

Box 8.F   Management of nausea and vomiting in palliative care (based on guidelines used at Sir Michael Sobell House, Oxford)

After clinical evaluation, document the most likely cause(s) of the nausea and vomiting in the patient's case notes.

Record severity, preferably using a formal rating scale.

Treat potentially reversible causes/exacerbating factors, e.g.

drugs	infection
constipation	cough
severe pain	hypercalcaemia *(correction is not always appropriate in a dying patient).*

Anxiety exacerbates nausea and vomiting from any cause and may need specific treatment, pharmacological and/or psychological.

Prescribe the first-line anti-emetic for the most likely main cause (see Table 8.12), both regularly and as needed.

If vomiting prevents enteral drug absorption or the patient is nauseated for most of the time, administer the anti-emetic parenterally, preferably SC by continuous infusion preceded by a stat dose or by regular injections through a butterfly cannula.

Optimize the dose of anti-emetic every 24 h, taking as needed use into account and the patient's own daily ratings of nausea and vomiting.

If little or no benefit after 24–48 h despite optimizing the dose, have you got the cause right?

- If no, change to the appropriate anti-emetic and optimize (see Table 8.12)
- If yes, provided the first-line anti-emetic has been optimized, add or substitute the second-line anti-emetic.

One-third of patients with nausea and vomiting need 2 anti-emetics.

Do not prescribe a prokinetic anti-emetic and an anticholinergic drug concurrently; the latter (including cyclizine) blocks the prokinetic action (see p.325).

Consider converting to an equivalent oral regimen after 72 h of good control with parenteral medication.

Continue the anti-emetic regimen indefinitely unless the cause is self-limiting.

Table 8.12 Drug management of nausea and vomiting in palliative care[a]

Cause	First-line drug	Stat dose	24 h range	Second-line drug	Stat dose	24 h range	Adjuncts
Gastric stasis	Metoclopramide[b] *prokinetic and dopamine antagonist*	10–20 mg	30–100 mg	Cisapride PO[b,c] (substitute) *prokinetic*	20 mg PO	20 mg b.d. PO	Antiflatulent, e.g. Asilone
Gastric irritation drugs radiotherapy	Metoclopramide[b]	10–20 mg	30–100 mg	Tropisetron[d] (substitute) *5HT$_3$ antagonist*	5 mg	5–10 mg	Proton pump inhibitor (e.g. lansoprazole) Misoprostol if NSAID-induced
Bowel obstruction without colic	Metoclopramide[b]	10–20 mg	40–100 mg	Dexamethasone (add) *corticosteroid*	8–12 mg IV	8–12 mg	Diamorphine (for background pain) Phosphate enema every 3–4 days to empty lower colon Faecal softener, e.g. docusate

continued

Table 8.12 Drug management of nausea and vomiting in palliative care[a]

Cause	First-line drug	Stat dose	24 h range	Second-line drug	Stat dose	24 h range	Adjuncts
Gastric stasis	Metoclopramide[b] *prokinetic and dopamine antagonist*	10–20 mg	30–100 mg	Cisapride PO[b,c] *(substitute) prokinetic*	20 mg PO	20 mg b.d. PO	Antiflatulent, e.g. Asilone
Gastric irritation drugs radiotherapy	Metoclopramide[b]	10–20 mg	30–100 mg	Tropisetron[d] *(substitute) 5HT₃ antagonist*	5 mg	5–10 mg	Proton pump inhibitor (e.g. lansoprazole) Misoprostol if NSAID-induced
Bowel obstruction without colic	Metoclopramide[b]	10–20 mg	40–100 mg	Dexamethasone (add) *corticosteroid*	8–12 mg IV	8–12 mg	Diamorphine (for background pain) Phosphate enema every 3–4 days to empty lower colon Faecal softener, e.g. docusate

continued

Table 8.12 continued

Cause	First-line drug	Stat dose	24 h range	Second-line drug	Stat dose	24 h range	Adjuncts
Raised intracranial pressure	Dexamethasone[e] plus	8–16 mg	8–16 mg	Cyclizine[b,g] (add if as needed doses continue to be required)			
	Cyclizine[b,g]	50 mg	Repeat q4h as needed		50 mg	100–200 mg	
Motion	Cyclizine	50 mg	Repeat q4h as needed				
	Hyoscine hydrobromide[b]	0.3 mg SL 0.4 mg SC	0.3 mg SL q.d.s. 0.8–1.2 mg SC				
Indeterminate	Metoclopramide[b]	10 mg	40–100 mg	Levomepromazine[b,h] (substitute)	6.25 mg	6.25–25 mg	Dexamethasone 8–16 mg/24 h[e] Tropisetron 5 mg o.d.[d,e]

a   most anti-emetics can be given SC; the dose of an anti-emetic is generally the same whether PO, SC or IV
b   anticholinergic drugs block the prokinetic effect of metoclopramide, cisapride and domperidone
c   cisapride is only available as a tablet; it is 2–4 times more potent than metoclopramide as a prokinetic
d   of value in situations where excess 5HT is released from enterochromaffin cells, e.g. chemotherapy, radiotherapy affecting the bowel, intestinal distension, renal failure
e   because of long duration of action, injection o.d. is preferable to SC infusion
f   reduces gastro-intestinal secretions
g   cyclizine lactate is irritant, and a more dilute infusate reduces inflammation around the butterfly cannula; use water to dilute because saline precipitates cyclizine; when used with diamorphine, do not exceed a concentration of cyclizine 20 mg/ml (see p.42)
h   less irritant if diluted in 0.9% saline; can be given by injection o.d.
i   for highly emetogenic chemotherapy, see BNF Sections 8.1 and 4.6.

Bowel obstruction

The focus here is on patients for whom available anticancer treatments have been exhausted.

Causes

- the cancer itself
- past treatment, e.g. adhesions, postradiation, ischaemic fibrosis
- associated with debility, e.g. constipation
- drugs (Table 8.13)
- an unrelated benign condition, e.g. strangulated hernia
- a combination of factors.

Table 8.13   Drugs used in palliative care contributing to obstruction

Drugs	Effects
Opioid	Cause hypersegmentation of the bowel
Anticholinergic (*see* p.352)	Interfere with parasympathetic nerve transmission
Anticoagulant	May cause paralytic ileus as the result of multiple intramural haemorrhages
Corticosteroid	Occasionally associated with mesenteric vascular occlusion

In consequence, bowel obstruction may be

- mechanical or functional, or both
- high or low, or both
- single or multiple sites
- partial or complete
- transient or persistent.

Clinical features

Abdominal pain associated with the underlying cancer is present in > 90% of cases. Vomiting occurs in 100% and intestinal colic in about 75%.[41,42] Distension is variable and bowel habit ranges from absolute constipation to diarrhoea. Bowel sounds vary from absent in adynamic obstructions to hyperactive and audible (borborygmi) in some dynamic obstructions. Tinkling bowel sounds are uncommon.

Management

Surgical

Surgical intervention is contra-indicated in each of the following circumstances

- previous laparotomy findings preclude the prospect of a successful intervention

- intra-abdominal carcinomatosis as evidenced by diffuse palpable intra-abdominal tumours

- massive ascites which re-accumulates rapidly after paracentesis.[43]

Surgical intervention should be considered if the following criteria are all fulfilled

- an easily reversible cause seems likely, e.g. postoperative adhesions or a single discrete neoplastic obstruction

- the patient's general condition is good, i.e. he does not have widely disseminated disease and has been independent and active

- the patient is willing to undergo surgery.

Medical

In patients in whom an operative approach is contra-indicated, it is generally possible to relieve symptoms adequately with drugs. A nasogastric tube and IV fluids are rarely necessary.

Eliminate pain and colic

- for constant background pain, administer diamorphine/morphine by continuous SC infusion using a portable syringe driver

- if the patient is experiencing colic:
      do not use a prokinetic drug
      discontinue bulk-forming, osmotic and stimulant laxatives

- if colic persists despite SC diamorphine/morphine, prescribe SC hyoscine butylbromide 60–120 mg/24 h in addition.

Eliminate nausea and reduce vomiting to once or twice a day

The choice of anti-emetic depends on whether the patient is experiencing colic. If yes, hyoscine butylbromide will have been started already. If no, the following sequence can be followed

- if passing flatus, a trial of SC metoclopramide 60–120 mg/24 h helps to determine whether the obstruction is more functional than mechanical[44]

- if not helpful, substitute SC cyclizine 100–150 mg/24 h

- if cyclizine fails, SC hyoscine butylbromide 60–120 mg/24 h should be tried because of its antisecretory properties[45]

- if there is persistent nausea (generally caused by toxic chemical factors), add haloperidol 5–10 mg/24 h

- alternatively, use SC levomepromazine 6.25–25 mg/24 h alone or in combination with hyoscine butylbromide[39]

- dexamethasone may be of benefit as a second anti-emetic, i.e. used in conjunction with metoclopramide or cyclizine.

Dexamethasone also helps in functional obstruction caused by perineural tumour.[19] In mechanical obstruction, dexamethasone is generally of limited benefit. Seeming benefit must be differentiated from spontaneous remission – seen in about one third of partially obstructed cancer patients.[46]

Because raised intraluminal pressure causes the release of 5HT from entero-chromaffin cells in the bowel, some patients benefit from a $5HT_3$-receptor antagonist.[47]

Octreotide 250–500 mcg/24 h can be used as an antisecretory agent instead of hyoscine butylbromide. This expensive somatostatin analogue has similar intestinal actions to hyoscine but no anticholinergic effects.[48] Published reports indicate that about 75% of patients benefit.[49,50] At Sobell House, octreotide is rarely used for obstruction because of its expense and a low success rate (about 20%) when used after the application of the above measures.

A venting percutaneous endoscopic gastrostomy is rarely necessary for symptom relief in patients with end-stage cancer.[51]

Relieve associated constipation

A phosphate enema should be given if constipation is a likely causal factor and a faecal softener prescribed, e.g. docusate tablets 100–200 mg b.d. If the small bowel only is affected, a colonic stimulant laxative can be used.

General

Inoperable patients managed by drug therapy should be encouraged to drink and eat small amounts of their favourite beverages and food. Some patients find that they can manage food best in the morning.

The use of anticholinergic drugs and diminished fluid intake often results in a dry mouth and thirst. These symptoms are generally relieved by conscientious mouth care (see p.159). A few ml of fluid every 30 min, possibly administered as a small ice cube, generally brings relief.[52] IV hydration is rarely needed.

Duodenum

Obstruction here is generally caused by cancer of the head of the pancreas. Most are functional and caused by disruption of duodenal peristalsis.

- try metoclopramide 60 mg/24 h by SC infusion

- if beneficial, optimize the dose and consider changing to cisapride 20 mg PO b.d. (see p.326)

- if the vomiting is made worse, it indicates mechanical obstruction; discontinue metoclopramide and prescribe an antihistaminic anti-emetic or hyoscine butylbromide instead (see p.201)

- if metoclopramide is of partial benefit, add dexamethasone 10–20 mg PO/ SC o.d. initially for 3 days; if improvement occurs it suggests that local tumour-induced inflammation may have been a causal factor

- if none of the above is of benefit, discuss the use of a nasogastric tube or a venting gastrostomy with the patient.

With a high bowel obstruction, it is generally not possible to stop vomiting completely. A practical goal is a much reduced frequency to 2–3 times/24 h.

Pylorus

Gastric cancer may cause mechanical pyloric obstruction. If surgery is contra-indicated

- prescribe hyoscine butylbromide 60–120 mg/24 h or octreotide 250–500 mcg/24 h by SC infusion

- try dexamethasone 10–20 mg PO/IM o.d. for 3 days

- discuss the use of a nasogastric tube or a venting gastrostomy with the patient.

Constipation

Description

Constipation is the evacuation of hard stools less frequently than is normal for an individual. Healthy people do not all defaecate daily.

- 5–7/week   75%
- < 3/week ⎫
- > 3/day   ⎬ 1%

Constipation can cause several serious secondary symptoms, e.g. overflow diarrhoea, urinary retention, bowel obstruction.

Causes

Table 8.14   Causes of constipation in advanced cancer

Related to cancer and/or debility	*Caused by drugs*
Hypercalcaemia	Opioids
Inactivity	NSAIDs
Poor nutrition	Anticholinergics
decreased intake	antihistaminic anti-emetics
low residue diet	phenothiazines
Poor fluid intake	tricyclics
Dehydration	5HT$_3$ antagonists
vomiting	Vincristine
polyuria	Diuretics
fever	dehydration
Weakness	hypokalaemia
Inability to reach toilet	
when urge to defaecate	

Management

Diet

- increase food intake
- add bran to diet

- increase fluid intake
- encourage fruit juices.

Exercise

- mobilize patient if possible.

Nursing measures

- prompt response to the patient's request to defaecate
- use a commode rather than a bedpan
- support the patient's feet on a foot stool to help brace the abdominal muscles
- raise the toilet seat and install hand rails in the patient's home to increase toilet independence.

Drugs

- stop or reduce the dose of constipating drugs
- use laxatives systematically (Box 8.G, Tables 8.15 and 8.16)
- the modal dose of co-danthrusate for patients not taking morphine is 1–2 capsules nocte; for those taking morphine 2 capsules b.d.

Rectal measures

- suppositories
- enemas
- manual removals.

One third of patients continue to need rectal measures despite oral laxatives. Some are elective, e.g. in paraplegics and the elderly and debilitated.

Box 8.G   Management of opioid-induced constipation

Ask about the patient's normal bowel habit and use of laxatives; record date of last bowel action.

Do a rectal examination if faecal impaction is suspected or if the patient reports diarrhoea or faecal incontinence (to exclude impaction with overflow).

For inpatients, record bowel actions each day in a Bowel Book.

Encourage fluids generally, and fruit juice and fruit specifically.

When an opioid is first prescribed, prescribe co-danthrusate[a] 1 capsule nocte prophylactically.

If already constipated, prescribe co-danthrusate 2 capsules nocte.

Adjust the dose every few days according to results, up to 3 capsules t.d.s.

If the patient prefers a liquid preparation, use co-danthrusate suspension; 5 ml is equivalent to 1 capsule.

If necessary, 'uncork' with suppositories, e.g. bisacodyl 10 mg and glycerine 4 g.

If suppositories are ineffective, administer a phosphate enema; possibly repeat the next day.

If the maximum dose of co-danthrusate is ineffective, reduce by half and add an osmotic laxative, e.g. lactulose 20–30 ml b.d.

If co-danthrusate causes abdominal cramps divide the daily dose into smaller, more frequent doses, e.g. change from co-danthrusate 2 capsules b.d. to 1 capsule q.d.s. or change to an osmotic laxative, e.g. lactulose 20–40 ml o.d.–t.d.s.

Lactulose may be preferable to co-danthrusate in patients with a history of irritable bowel syndrome or of colic with other colonic stimulants, e.g. senna.

Sometimes it is appropriate to optimize a patient's existing bowel regimen, rather than change automatically to co-danthrusate.

---

a   in USA, use Peri-Colace (casanthranol 30 mg + docusate sodium 100 mg) capsules instead.

Table 8.15 Classification of laxatives

Bulk-forming drugs (fibre)

Bran
Methylcellulose
Mucilloids
    psyllium (Metamucil)
    ispaghula (Isogel, Fybogel, Regulan)
    sterculia (Normacol)

Lubricants

Liquid paraffin/mineral oil

Salines

Magnesium salts
Sodium sulphate
Sodium phosphate

Osmotic agents (small bowel flushers)

Lactulose
Sorbitol (30–70%)
Mannitol (20%

Contact laxatives (peristaltic stimulants)

1 Small and large bowel

Bile salts
Ricinoleic acid
  (in castor oil) } surface wetting agents (faecal softeners)
Docusate[a]

2 Mainly large bowel

Polyphenolics
  phenolphthalein
  bisacodyl
  sodium picosulphate
Synthetic anthracene
  danthron

3 Large bowel only

Natural anthracenes
  senna
  casanthranol (not UK)
  cascara (not UK)

a   in typical doses, i.e. 100–200 mg b.d., docusate is predominantly a faecal softener.

Table 8.16 Composition of laxatives (UK)

Bulk-forming drugs

Fybogel (sachet)
Regulan (sachet) } Ispaghula husk 3.4–6.4 g
Normacol granules   Sterculia 6.2 g/10 g
Normacol plus granules   Sterculia 6.2 g/10 g +
Celevac tablet   frangula 800 mg/10 g
                           Methylcellulose 500 mg

Salines and lubricants

Milk of magnesia suspension (5 ml)   Magnesium hydroxide 350 mg
Liquid paraffin and magnesium   Magnesium hydroxide mixture BP
   hydroxide emulsion BP (10 ml)   7.5 ml + liquid paraffin 2.5 ml
Epsom salts
   crystals (5 ml)
   solution (10 ml) } Magnesium sulphate 4 g

Osmotic agents

Lactulose syrup 3.35 g/5 ml

Surface wetting agents

Docusate solution 50 mg/5 ml
Docusate tablet 100 mg

Contact laxatives

Standardized senna tablet 7.5 mg
Bisacodyl tablet 5 mg
Bisacodyl suppository 5 mg, 10 mg
Sodium picosulphate syrup 5 mg/5 ml
Co-danthrusate suspension (5 ml)/capsule Danthron 50 mg + docusate 60 mg
Co-danthramer suspension (5 ml)/capsule   Danthron 25 mg + poloxamer 200 mg
Co-danthramer strong capsule   Danthron 37.5 mg + poloxamer 500 mg
Co-danthramer strong suspension (5 ml)   Danthron 75 mg + poloxamer 1 g

Faecal impaction

Definition

Faecal impaction is the lodging of faeces in the rectum (90%) or in the colon, occasionally as far back as the caecum.

Pathogenesis

Incomplete evacuation leads to cumulation of faeces in the rectum. The faeces become very firm because fluid is absorbed from them while they remain in contact with the bowel mucosa. Additional faecal material increases the size of the mass so that it becomes physically impossible for it to be evacuated. Bacterial liquefaction of more proximal faeces may result in overflow diarrhoea and faecal leakage.

Sometimes a soft impaction occurs. This is more likely if the impaction occurs despite the use of a bulk-forming drug or a faecal softener.

Causes

The causes of faecal impaction are similar to those of constipation (Table 8.17).

Table 8.17   Causes of faecal impaction in advanced cancer

Caused by cancer	Related to cancer and/or debility
Tumour blocking passage of solid faeces	Weakness Being bedbound Mental impairment
Caused by drugs	Concurrent causes
Aluminium antacids Barium Anticholinergics Opioids etc.	Anal stricture Anal fissure

Clinical features

The patient complains of constipation or of the frequent passage of small quantities of fluid faeces together with some or all of the following

• rectal discharge

- spasmodic rectal pain – may be agonizing
- abdominal colic
- abdominal distension
- nausea and vomiting.

A very ill or elderly patient may develop an agitated delirium.

Evaluation

A high level of suspicion is helpful in the diagnosis of faecal impaction and overflow diarrhoea. The patient may indicate that he has become progressively more constipated but then, 'They suddenly become loose. The trouble is I can't tell when my bowels are going to act – I have no warning.'

Abdominal examination often reveals hard faecal material in the descending and sigmoid colons; the transverse and ascending colons may also be involved. A dilated caecum may be noted. Although rectal examination generally confirms the presence of a large faecal mass, an empty rectum cannot rule out a high impaction.

Management

Soft faeces

- bisacodyl 10–20 mg PR o.d. until there is a negative response
- contact with the rectal mucosa is essential for absorption
- give PO if mucosal contact impossible.

Hard faeces

- give an arachis oil retention enema (130 ml) overnight
- premedicate with IV midazolam or diazepam, and disrupt the faecal mass by finger manipulation and remove piecemeal
- rectal contents can be further softened by a retention enema of docusate, e.g. 300 mg in 100 ml (i.e. diluted oral syrup) or a proprietary docusate micro-enema (these contain 90–120 mg)

- follow the next day with a high phosphate enema, i.e. use a 45 cm plastic catheter attached to the enema-giving set

- prescribe oral laxatives to prevent recurrence.

Diarrhoea

Description

Diarrhoea is an increase in the frequency of defaecation and/or fluidity of the faeces. If severe, it may manifest as faecal incontinence.

Causes

There are many potential causes (Table 8.18). Three common ones are

- laxative overdose

- faecal impaction and overflow diarrhoea

- partial bowel obstruction.[33]

Diarrhoea is common in AIDS; a pathogen (or pathogens) is identifiable in about half of the cases.[53]

Other relatively common causes include

- radiation enteritis

- drugs (Table 8.19)

- steatorrhea.

Steatorrhoea is often called diarrhoea by the patient.

Cholegenic diarrhoea

Active absorption of bile acids occurs mainly in the distal ileum. Nonabsorbed bile acids are metabolized in the colon by bacterial enzymes to form unconjugated α-dihydroxy bile acids which stimulate fluid and electrolyte secretion. This results in cholegenic diarrhoea which is often explosive and watery, and poorly responsive to standard antidiarrhoeals.

Table 8.18 Causes of diarrhoea in advanced cancer

Mechanical causes	Caused by treatment
Overflow	Drugs (see Table 8.19)
obstruction	Radiotherapy
faecal impaction	Chemotherapy
Short bowel	5-fluoro-uracil
bowel resection	mitomycin
colostomy	methotrexate
ileostomy	cytosine arabinoside
ileocolic fistula	doxorubicin
	etoposide
Functional causes	asparaginase
	Coeliac axis plexus block[54]
Diet	
bran	*Concurrent causes*
fruit	
curry	Gastro-enteritis
alcohol	Irritable bowel syndrome
Steatorrhoea	Ulcerative colitis
pancreatic cancer	Diabetes mellitus
obstructive jaundice	Heart failure[55]
blind loop syndrome	
Visceral neuropathy	
paraneoplastic	
coeliac axis plexus block	
lumbar sympathectomy	
Carcinoid syndrome	

Loss of the ileocaecal valve may lead to bacterial invasion of the small intestine and more severe diarrhoea. The loss of small bowel hormonal inhibitors of gastrin secretion may lead to increased gastric acid and increased denaturation of pancreatic enzymes – adding steatorrhoea to the cholegenic diarrhoea.

Pseudomembranous colitis

Pseudomembranous colitis is an uncommon complication of antibiotic therapy (Table 8.20). Symptoms generally begin within 1 week of starting antibiotic therapy or shortly after stopping, but may occur up to 1 month later. It is caused by colonization of the bowel by *Clostridium difficile* and the production of toxins A and B which cause mucosal damage.

Table 8.19   Drug-induced diarrhoea in advanced cancer

Common	Occasional
Laxatives	Cisapride
Misoprostol	NSAIDs
Antacids	Oestrogens
magnesium salts	diethylstilbestrol > 3 mg/day
Antibiotics	Theophylline
erythromycin	Anticholinesterases
penicillins	neostigmine
sulphonamides	Hypoglycaemics
tetracyclines	sulphonylureas, e.g. chlorpropramide
(see also Table 8.20)	biguanides, e.g. metformin
Iron	Sorbitol[b]
Fenamates	Caffeine
SSRIs	
Overflow[a]	
Opioids	
Anticholinergics	
Aluminium hydroxide	

a   all drugs which predispose to constipation may lead to overflow diarrhoea
b   a nonabsorbable disaccharide used as a sweetener in 'sugar free' liquid medicines.

Table 8.20   Pseudomembranous colitis

	Causal antibiotics	
Clinical features	Most prevalent	Highest incidence
Explosive foul-smelling watery diarrhoea + mucus +/– blood	Ampicillin	Clindamycin
	Amoxycillin	Lincomycin
Abdominal pain	Cephalosporins	
Tenderness	Ciprofloxacin	
Fever		

C. difficile is strongly anaerobic and difficult to culture. Treatment is based on the history and clinical features. Faecal tests to detect *C. difficile* toxins serve to confirm. If in doubt, endoscopy and rectal biopsy are of value, although a trial of therapy is more practical

- metronidazole 400 mg PO q8h for 10 days (cheap)
- vancomycin 125 mg PO q6h for 10 days (expensive).

About 20% of patients relapse, most within 3 weeks. Mild relapses often resolve spontaneously. Repeated relapses require prolonged treatment with slowly decreasing doses of vancomycin.[56]

Evaluation

A carefully elicited history and clinical examination is often sufficient to determine the most likely cause. A careful review of medication is important. This will generally demonstrate if too much laxative is the cause.

If the history and examination do not point to a likely cause, faecal microscopy and culture are possibly indicated.

Management

- review medication, including laxatives
- review diet (Table 8.21)
- prescribe specific antidote (Table 8.22)
- prescribe a nonspecific antidiarrhoeal drug (Table 8.22)
- consider antibiotic treatment if cause infective or if bacterial overgrowth seems likely.

Table 8.21   Laxative foods

Raw fruit (fresh or dried)	Coleslaw
Nuts	Sauerkraut
Greens	Spicy foods
Beans	Wholegrain cereals
Lentils	Wholemeal foods
Onion	

Table 8.22 Drugs for treating diarrhoea

Disease specific	Nonspecific

Acute radiation enteritis
  NSAID
  cholestyramine
	Absorbants
	  hydrophilic bulking agents
	  pectin

Steatorrhoea
  pancreatin supplements
	Adsorbants
	  kaolin
	  attapulgite

Cholegenic diarrhoea
  cholestyramine (anion exchange
    resin)
	chalk
	
	Mucosal PG inhibitors
	  aspirin

Carcinoid syndrome cyproheptadine	bismuth subsalicylate

Pseudomembranous colitis
  metronidazole
  vancomycin
	Opioids
	  codeine
	  morphine
	  diphenoxylate

Ulcerative colitis
  sulphasalazine
  mesalazine
  corticosteroids
	loperamide
	
	Somatostatin analogues
	  octreotide

Infection appropriate antibiotic	

Loperamide is about 3 times more potent than diphenoxylate and 50 times more potent than codeine. It is longer acting and generally needs to be given only b.d. The following regimens are approximately equivalent:

loperamide	2 mg b.d.
diphenoxylate	2.5 mg (in Lomotil) q.d.s.
codeine phosphate	60 mg t.d.s.–q.d.s.

Kaolin and morphine mixture BP is a useful alternative preparation.

Loperamide 4 mg is the typical initial dose for acute diarrhoea, followed by 2 mg after each loose bowel action. It is uncommon to need more than 16 mg/24 h but doses up to 32 mg/24 h can be used.

In AIDS, morphine PO or diamorphine by SC infusion may be necessary to achieve control. These drugs have both peripheral and central constipating effects, whereas loperamide acts only peripherally.

Pancreatic enzyme replacement

Pancreatin is a standardized preparation of animal lipase, protease and amylase. Pancreatin hydrolyses fats to glycerol and fatty acids, changes protein into proteoses and derived substances, and converts starch into dextrin and sugars.

It is given by mouth in pancreatic deficiency in daily doses of ≤ 8 g in divided doses. Because 90% of administered pancreatin is destroyed in the stomach by gastric acid, an H_2-receptor antagonist or proton pump inhibitor should be prescribed concurrently.

Preparations of choice

- Creon capsules – each contains enteric-coated granules providing, inter alia, lipase 8000 units. Initially give 1–2 capsules with each meal, either whole or capsule contents added to fluid or soft food which must be swallowed without chewing; titrate dose upwards until a satisfactory response is obtained

- Creon 25 000 capsules – each contains enteric-coated granules providing, inter alia, lipase 25 000 units. Initially give 1 capsule with each meal, taken as above.

Fibrotic strictures of the colon have occurred in children under 13 years old with cystic fibrosis using other high-strength pancreatin preparations (Nutrizym 22, Pancreatin HL). None has been reported in adults or in patients without cystic fibrosis, or in patients of any age receiving Creon 25 000.

Rectal discharge

Causes

- patulous anus
- haemorrhoids
- faecal impaction and overflow
- following bowel evacuation after laxative suppositories (transient)
- rectal tumour
- radiation coloproctitis
- fistula:
    ileorectal
    rectovesical.

Clinical features

- discharge

- maceration

- pruritus

- malodour.

Management

Correct or modify cause

- faecal disimpaction (*see* p.208)

- reduce tumour size:
    radiation therapy
    fulguration (surgical diathermy)
    transanal resection
    LASER treatment

- reduce peritumour or postradiation inflammation:
    prednisolone suppositories 5 mg b.d.
    prednisolone retention enema 20 mg every 2–3 days.

Protection of skin of perineum and genitalia

- do not use toilet paper

- wash anal area with a soft cloth after each bowel action and as necessary

- use water only; do not use soap

- pat dry with soft cloth

- if above measures do not keep the area dry, protect the skin with a barrier, e.g. Morhulin ointment (zinc oxide 38% and cod-liver oil 11% in wool fat and paraffin) or Comfeel barrier cream

- monitor carefully for small blisters suggestive of fungal infection; treat with clotrimazole 1% solution or cream b.d.–t.d.s.

- use cotton underclothes and change at least o.d.

If very inflamed, consider applying clioquinol-hydrocortisone cream or hydro-cortisone spray b.d.–t.d.s.

Pruritus

If anal hygiene fails to relieve pruritus ani, prescribe an antihistamine.

Ascites

Severe ascites cause a range of symptoms (Table 8.23).

Table 8.23 Clinical features of ascites

Abdominal distension	Acid reflux
Abdominal discomfort/pain	Nausea and vomiting
Inability to sit upright	Leg oedema
Early satiety	Dyspnoea
Dyspepsia	

Pathogenesis

- generally associated with peritoneal metastases
- subphrenic lymphatics become blocked by tumour infiltration
- increased peritoneal permeability
- hyperaldosteronism, possibly secondary to reduced extracellular fluid volume, causes sodium retention and further feeds the ascitic process
- liver metastases leading to hypo-albuminaemia and, sometimes, portal hypertension.

Management

Chemotherapy

- systemic
- intraperitoneal.

These options are not discussed here.

Diuretics

Spironolactone is the key to success because it antagonizes aldosterone (Table 8.24).[57] Two thirds of patients are controlled on spironolactone 300 mg o.d. or less.[58]

The dose of the loop diuretic should be reduced once a satisfactory result is achieved.

Failure with diuretic therapy generally relates to

• gastric intolerance (spironolactone)

• too small a dose of spironolactone

• failure to use concomitant loop diuretic in resistant cases.

Table 8.24   Diuretic treatment of malignant ascites

		Loop diuretic		
	Spironolactone	Furosemide	or	Bumetanide
Day 1	100–200 mg o.d.	–		–
Day 7	200–300 mg o.d.	40 mg		1 mg
Day 14	200 mg b.d.	80 mg		2 mg

Paracentesis

Paracentesis is appropriate for patients with a tense distended abdomen and for those who cannot tolerate spironolactone tablets. The aim is to remove as much fluid as possible using an IV cannula or suprapubic catheter. Patients obtain short term relief even after the removal of only 2 l.

Paracentesis can be repeated if diuretics do not prevent re-accumulation. For patients who have had difficulties in the past, a paracentesis with ultrasound guidance should be considered.

Peritoneovenous shunt

This is a theoretical option in a patient who is relatively fit but cannot tolerate diuretic therapy.[59] Shunts are not often used in malignant ascites. When used, they may function satisfactorily for only a few weeks or months.[60]

References

1 Kusler DL and Rambur BA (1992) Treatment for radiation-induced xerostomia: an innovative study. *Cancer Nursing.* **15**: 191–195.

2 Anonymous (1994) Oral pilocarpine for xerostomia. *Medical Letter.* **34**: 76.

3 Kim JH *et al.* (1985) A clinical study of benzydamine for the treatment of radiotherapy induced mucositis of the oropharynx. *International Journal of Tissue Reaction.* **7**: 215–218.

4 NIH Consensus Development Conference Statement (1989) Oral complications of cancer therapies: diagnosis, prevention and treatment. *NIH Consensus Statement.* **7**: 1–11.

5 Mueller BA *et al.* (1995) Mucositis management practices for hospitalized patients: National survey results. *Journal of Pain and Symptom Management.* **10**: 510–520.

6 Burgess JA *et al.* (1990) Pharmacological management of recurrent oral mucosal ulceration. *Drugs.* **39**: 54–65.

7 Moertel CG *et al.* (1974) Corticosteroid therapy for preterminal gastrointestinal cancer. *Cancer.* **33**: 1607–1609.

8 Bruera E *et al.* (1985) Action of oral methylprednisolone in terminal cancer patients: a prospective randomized double-blind study. *Cancer Treatment Reports.* **69**: 751–754.

9 Downer S *et al.* (1993) A double blind placebo controlled trial of medroxyprogesterone acetate (MPA) in cancer cachexia. *British Journal of Cancer.* **67**: 1102–1105.

10 Burge F (1993) Dehydration symptoms of palliative care cancer patients. *Journal of Pain and Symptom Management.* **8**: 454–464.

11 Meares CJ (1994) Terminal dehydration: a review. *American Journal of Hospice and Palliative Care.* **11** (3): 10–14.

12 Dunphy K *et al.* (1995) Rehydration in palliative and terminal care: if not – why not? *Palliative Medicine.* **9**: 221–228.

13 Fainsinger RL *et al.* (1994) the use of hypodermoclysis for rehydration in terminally ill cancer patients. *Journal of Pain and Symptom Management.* **9**: 298–302.

14 Constans T *et al.* (1991) Hypodermoclysis in dehydrated elderly patients: local effects with and without hyaluronidase. *Journal of Palliative Care.* **7** (2): 10–12.

15 Bruera E *et al.* (1995) Changing pattern of agitated impaired mental status in patients with advanced cancer: association with cognitive monitoring, hydration, and opioid rotation. *Journal of Pain and Symptom Management.* **10**: 287–291.

16 Bruera E and Higginson I (1996) *Cachexia-Anorexia in Cancer Patients.* Oxford University Press, Oxford.

17 Logemann JA (1983) *Evaluation and treatment of swallowing disorders.* College Hill Press, San Diego.

18 Twycross RG and Regnard C (1997) Dysphagia, dyspepsia and hiccup. In: D Doyle, GW Hanks and N MacDonald (eds) *Oxford Textbook of Palliative Medicine.* Oxford University Press, Oxford. (in press)

19 Carter RL *et al.* (1982) Pain and dysphagia in patients with squamous carcinomas of the head and neck: the role of perineural spread. *Journal of the Royal Society of Medicine.* **72**: 598–606.

20 Murray FE *et al.* (1988) Palliative laser therapy for advanced esophageal carcinoma: an alternative perspective. *American Journal of Gastroenterology.* **83**: 816–820.

21 Carter R *et al.* (1992) Laser recanalization versus endoscopic intubation in the palliation of malignant dysphagia: a randomized prospective study. *British Journal of Surgery.* **79**: 1167–1170.

22 Lewis-Jones CM *et al.* (1995) Laser therapy in the palliation of dysphagia in oesophageal malignancy. *Palliative Medicine.* **9**: 327–330.

23 Nwokolo CU *et al.* (1994) Palliation of malignant dysphagia by ethanol induced tumour necrosis. *Gut.* **35**: 299–303.

24 Chung SCS *et al.* (1994) Palliation of malignant oesophageal obstruction by endoscopic alcohol injection. *Endoscopy.* **26**: 275–277.

25 Moran BJ and Frost RA (1992) Percutaneous endoscopic gastrostomy in 41 patients: indications and clinical outcome. *Journal of the Royal Society of Medicine.* **85**: 320–321.

26 McCamish MA and Crocker NJ (1993) Enteral and parenteral nutrition support of terminally ill patients: practical and ethical perspectives. *The Hospice Journal.* **9**: 107–129.

27 Bozzetti F (1996) Guidelines on artificial nutrition versus hydration in terminal cancer patients. *Nutrition.* **12**: 163–167.

28 van Berkel AM *et al.* (1996) Wallstents for metastatic biliary obstruction. *Endoscopy.* **28**: 418–421.

29 Feins RH *et al.* (1996) Palliation of inoperable oesophageal carcinoma with the Wallstent endoprosthesis. *Annals of Thoracic Surgery.* **62**: 1603–1607.

30 Rabeneck L *et al.* (1997) Ethically justified, clinically comprehensive guidelines for percutaneous endoscopic gastrostomy tube placement. *Lancet.* **349**: 496–498.

31 Mandel L and Tamari K (1995) Sialorrhea and gastroesophageal reflux. *Journal of the American Dental Association.* **126**: 1537–1541.

32 Talley NJ *et al.* (1991) Functional dyspepsia: a classification with guidelines for diagnosis and management. *Gastroenterology International.* **4** (4): 145–160.

33 Twycross R and Lack SA (1986) *Control of Alimentary Symptoms in Far-Advanced Cancer.* Churchill Livingstone, Edinburgh.

34 Nelson KA *et al.* (1993) Assessment of upper gastrointestinal motility in the cancer-associated dyspepsia syndrome (CADS). *Journal of Palliative Care.* **9** (1): 27–31.

35 Armes PJ *et al.* (1992) A study to investigate the incidence of early satiety in patients with advanced cancer. *British Journal of Cancer.* **65**: 481–484.

36 Bruera E *et al.* (1987) Chronic nausea and anorexia in advanced cancer patients: A possible role for autonomic dysfunction. *Journal of Pain and Symptom Management.* **2**: 19–21.

37 Bruera E *et al.* (1986) Study of cardiovascular autonomic insufficiency in advanced cancer patients. *Cancer Treatment Reports.* **70**: 1383–1387.

38 Levitt M (1983) Gastrointestinal gas and abdominal symptoms. *Practical Gastroenterology.* **7**: 6–12.

39 Twycross RG *et al.* (1997) The use of low dose levomepromazine (methotrimeprazine) in the management of nausea and vomiting. *Progress in Palliative Care.* **5** (2): 49–53.

40 Barnes J and Barnes N (1991) Effective management of nausea and vomiting. *Prescriber.* **October 19**: 29–34.

41 Baines M *et al.* (1985) Medical management of intestinal obstruction in patients with advanced malignant disease: a clinical and pathological study. *Lancet.* **2**: 990–993.

42 Baines M (1987) Medical management of intestinal obstruction. *Bailliere's Clinical Oncology.* **1** (2): Bailliere Tindall, London.

43 Krebs HB and Goplerud DR (1987) Mechanical intestinal obstruction in patients with gynecologic disease: A review of 368 patients. *American Journal of Obstetrics and Gynecology.* **157**: 577–583.

44 Isbister WH *et al.* (1990) Nonoperative management of malignant intestinal obstruction. *Journal of the Royal College of Surgeons, Edinburgh.* **35**: 369–372.

45 DeConno F *et al.* (1991) Continuous subcutaneous infusion of hyoscine butyl-bromide reduces secretions in patients with gastrointestinal obstruction. *Journal of Pain and Symptom Management.* **6**: 484–486.

46 Glass RL and LeDuc RJ (1973) Small intestinal obstruction from peritoneal carcinomatosis. *American Journal of Surgery.* **125**: 316–317.

47 Huchison SMW *et al.* (1995) Increased serotonin excretion in patients with ovarian carcinoma and intestinal obstruction. *Palliative Medicine.* **9**: 67–68.

48 Fallon MT (1994) The physiology of somatostatin and its synthetic analogue, octreotide. *European Journal of Palliative Care.* **1**: 20–22.

49 Khoo D *et al.* (1994) Palliation of malignant intestinal obstruction using octreotide. *European Journal of Cancer.* **30A**: 28–30.

50 Riley J and Fallon MT (1994) Octreotide in terminal malignant obstruction of the gastrointestinal tract. *European Journal of Palliative Care.* **1**: 23–25.

51 Ashby MA *et al.* (1991) Percutaneous gastrostomy as a venting procedure in palliative care. *Palliative Medicine.* **5**: 147–150.

52 Guyton AC (1971) *Basic human physiology: normal function and mechanisms of disease.* WB Saunders, Philadelphia, 1971.

53 Rolston KVI *et al.* (1989) Diarrhoea in patients infected with the human immuno-deficiency virus. *American Journal of Medicine.* **86**: 137–138.

54 Dean AP and Reed WD (1991) Diarrhoea – an unrecognised hazard of coeliac plexus block. *Australian and New Zealand Journal of Medicine.* **21**: 47–48.

55 McCarthy M (1996) Dying from heart disease. *Journal of the Royal College of Physicians of London.* **30**: 325–328.

56 Anonymous (1995) Antibiotic-induced diarrhoea. *Drug and Therapeutics Bulletin.* **33** (3): 23–24.

57 Fogel MR *et al.* (1981) Diuresis in the ascitic patient: a randomized controlled trial of three regimens. *Journal of Clinical Gastroenterology* **3** (Suppl 1): 73–80.

58 Greenway B *et al.* (1982) Control of malignant ascites with spironolactone. *British Journal of Surgery.* **69**: 441–442.

59 Osterlee J (1980) Peritoneovenous shunting for ascites in cancer patients. *British Journal of Surgery.* **67**: 663–666.

60 Soderlund C (1986) Denver peritoneovenous shunting for malignant or cirrhotic ascites. A prospective consecutive series. *Scandinavian Journal of Gastroenterology.* **21**: 1167–1172.

9 Urinary symptoms

Useful definitions · Urinary bladder innervation
Frequency and urgency · Bladder spasms
Hesitancy · Discoloured urine

Useful definitions

Frequency	Passage of urine seven or more times during the day and twice or more at night.
Urgency	A strong and sudden desire to void.
Urge incontinence	The involuntary loss of urine associated with a strong desire to void.
Detrusor instability	Detrusor contracts uninhibitedly and causes: diurnal frequency, nocturnal frequency, urgency, urge incontinence — increasing severity. (Detrusor instability is the second most common cause of urinary incontinence in women.)
Stress incontinence	The involuntary loss of urine associated with coughing, sneezing, laughing and lifting.
Genuine stress incontinence (Urethral sphincter incompetence)	The involuntary loss of urine when the intravesical pressure exceeds maximum urethral pressure in the *absence of detrusor activity*. The fault always lies in the sphincter mechanisms of the bladder, and is associated with multiparity, postmenopause and posthysterectomy. One or more of the following features will be present: descent of urethrovesical junction outside intra-abdominal zone of pressure; decrease in urethral pressure due to loss of urethral wall elasticity and contractility; short functional length of urethra. (Urethral sphincter incompetence is the most common cause of urinary incontinence in women.)

continued

| Dysuria | Pain during and/or after micturition. Often urethral in origin (a burning sensation) but may be caused by bladder spasm (intense suprapubic and urethral pain), or both. |

Urinary bladder innervation

'You pee with your parasympathetics. You stop with your sympathetics.'

The sphincter relaxes when the detrusor (bladder muscle) contracts, and vice versa (Table 9.1). Thus anticholinergic (antimuscarinic) drugs not only cause contraction of the bladder neck sphincter but also relax the detrusor.

Detrusor sensitivity is

- increased by PGs
- decreased by COX inhibitors, i.e. NSAIDs.

The urethral sphincter is an additional voluntary mechanism innervated by the pudendal nerve (S2–4).

The urethra, derived embryologically from the urogenital sinus, is sensitive in the female to oestrogen and progesterone. Postmenopausal urge incontinence and frequency is sometimes helped by the prescription of an oestrogen, either topically or orally. Oestrogens do not improve stress incontinence.

Morphine and other opioids have several effects on bladder function (Table 9.2). These are generally asymptomatic. Occasionally hesitancy or retention occurs.

Table 9.1 Autonomic innervation of urinary bladder

| Innervation | Mediator | Effect on | |
		Sphincter	Vault
Sympathetic (T10–12, L1)	Norepinephrine	Contracts (α)	Relaxes (β)
Parasympathetic (S2–4)	Acetylcholine	Relaxes	Contracts

Table 9.2 Morphine and the urinary tract

Bladder sensation decreased

Sphincter tone *increased*

Detrusor tone *increased*

Ureteric tone and amplitude of contractions increased

Frequency and urgency

Incidence

The incidence of frequency, urgency and urge incontinence in cancer patients, or in those with urinary tract cancers, is not known. Frequency is often associated with urgency, which may result in urge incontinence.

Causes

The causes of frequency and urgency overlap with those of urge incontinence (Table 9.3). Tiaprofenic acid (a NSAID) can cause severe cystitis with haematuria

Table 9.3 Causes of urgency and incontinence

Caused by cancer	*Related to cancer and/or debility*
Pain	Infective cystitis
Hypercalcaemia (causes polyuria)	
Intravesical ⎱ mechanical	*Concurrent causes*
Extravesical ⎰ irritation	
Bladder spasms	Idiopathic detrusor instability
Sacral plexopathy	Central neurological disease
	poststroke
Caused by treatment	multiple sclerosis
	dementia
Radiation cystitis	Uraemia ⎱
Cyclophosphamide cystitis	Diabetes mellitus ⎰ cause polyuria
Drugs	Diabetes insipidus
diuretics	
tiaprofenic acid	

as a direct toxic effect of the drug and/or its metabolites on the bladder. Presentation is generally several months, or even years, after starting treatment with tiaprofenic acid.[1,2]

The precipitating factor in urge incontinence is delayed micturition relative to need. Delay is associated with

- weakness and difficulty in getting to a commode
- disinterest:
    depression
    dejection
- lack of awareness:
    confusion
    drowsiness.

The differential diagnosis includes

- genuine stress incontinence
- retention with overflow
- urinary fistula
- flaccid sphincter (presacral plexopathy).

Management

Explanation

Treat reversible causes

- reduce or change diuretic
- stop tiaprofenic acid
- treat infective cystitis with antibiotic or cranberry juice.

Cranberry juice acidifies urine and inhibits bacterial adherence to the bladder mucosa.[3] 180 ml b.d. of 33% cranberry juice is of proven benefit. The addition of ascorbic acid (vitamin C) is not necessary, although sometimes recommended.

Nondrug measures

- regular time-contingent voiding, e.g. every 1–3 h
- proximity to toilet

- ready availability of bottle or commode
- rapid response by nurses to patient's request for help.

Drugs

- anticholinergics are the drugs of choice even though treatment may be limited by associated unwanted anticholinergic effects (*see* p.352):
    oxybutynin 2.5–5 mg b.d.–q.d.s.; also has a topical anaesthetic effect on the bladder mucosa[4]
    amitriptyline 25–50 mg nocte
    propantheline 15 mg b.d.–t.d.s.
- sympathomimetics, e.g. terbutaline 5 mg t.d.s.
- musculotropic drugs, e.g. flavoxate 200–400 mg q.d.s.
- NSAIDs, e.g.
    flurbiprofen 50–100 mg b.d.
    naproxen 250–500 mg b.d.
- topical analgesics, e.g. phenazopyridine 100–200 mg t.d.s. (not available in the UK)
- vasopressin/antidiuretic hormone analogues, e.g. desmopressin 200–400 mcg PO nocte, are often of value in refractory troublesome nocturia.[5] Monitor plasma sodium concentration; hyponatraemia is a possible complication.

Bladder spasms

Bladder (detrusor) spasms are transient, often excruciating, sensations felt in the suprapubic region and urethra. They are generally secondary to irritation of the trigone.

Causes

Bladder spasms may relate to local cancer or other factors (Table 9.4).

Table 9.4   Causes of bladder spasms

Caused by cancer	*Related to cancer and/or debility*
Intravesical ⎫ Extravesical ⎭ irritation	Anxiety Infective cystitis Indwelling catheter:
Caused by treatment	mechanical irritation by catheter balloon catheter sludging with partial retention
Radiation fibrosis	

Management

Explanation

Treat reversible causes

Treatment options for reversible causes are listed in Table 9.5.

Analgesics

Analgesics should be used to relieve background pain.

Drugs to reduce detrusor sensitivity

- anticholinergics are the drugs of choice
    oxybutynin 2.5–5 mg b.d.–q.d.s. ⎫
    amitriptyline 25–50 mg nocte   ⎬ same as for urgency
    propantheline 15 mg b.d.–t.d.s. ⎭

- hyoscine (Quick Kwells) 0.3 mg b.d.–q.d.s. SL

- hyoscyamine (twice as potent as hyoscine; not available in the UK), e.g.
    0.15 mg b.d.–q.d.s. or m/r 0.375 mg b.d.

- belladonna and opium suppositories (B & O Supprettes USA) up to hourly:
    each B & O Supprette contains either 30 mg (No. 15A) or 60 mg (No.
    16A) of powdered opium and approximately 0.2 mg of belladonna
    alkaloids

- flavoxate 100–200 mg t.d.s.–q.d.s. (a weak detrusor relaxant)

- NSAIDs, e.g.
    flurbiprofen 50–100 mg b.d.
    naproxen 250–500 mg b.d.

- phenazopyridine 100–200 mg t.d.s. (a topical transitional cell analgesic;
    not available in the UK).

Table 9.5   Treatment of reversible causes of bladder spasms

Cause	Treatment

Infection (cystitis)	Bladder washouts (if catheterized)
	 Change indwelling catheter
	 Intermittent catheterization q4h–q6h
	 Encourage oral fluids
	 Cranberry juice
	 Urinary antiseptics (effective only in acid urine)
	     hexamine hippurate
	     hexamine mandelate
	 Antibiotics
	     systemic
	     by instillation

Catheter irritation	Change catheter Reduce volume of balloon

Catheter sludging	Bladder washouts
	     tap water
	     saline
	     chlorhexidine and benzocaine (Hibitane)[a]
	     solution G[b]
	 Continuous bladder irrigation

a   there is no evidence that chlorhexidine is better than saline or tap water; its use may cause the emergence of resistant bacterial strains

b   cost about £2.50 per sachet and contains citric acid, sodium bicarbonate etc.; use if troublesome urinary sediment causes repeated catheter blockage despite saline washouts.

Interrupt pain pathways

• coeliac axis plexus block

• lumbar sympathetic block.

Hesitancy

Definition

Hesitancy is a prolonged delay between attempting and achieving micturition.

Causes

The causes of hesitancy and retention are shown in Table 9.6.

Table 9.6   Causes of hesitancy and retention

Caused by cancer	*Related to cancer and/or debility*
Malignant enlargement of prostate	Loaded rectum
Infiltration of bladder neck	Inability to stand to micturate
Presacral plexopathy	Generalized weakness
Spinal cord compression	
	Concurrent causes
Caused by treatment	
	Benign enlargement of prostate
Anticholinergic drugs (*see* p.352)	
Morphine (occasionally)	
Spinal analgesia (particularly with	
bupivacaine)	
Intrathecal nerve block	

Management

Explanation

Treat reversible causes

Treatment options for reversible causes of hesitancy are listed in Table 9.7.

Table 9.7   Treatment of reversible causes of hesitancy

Causes	Treatment
Anticholinergic drugs	Modify drug regimen if possible
Loaded rectum	Suppositories ⎫ Enema ⎬ → maintenance laxative regimen Manual removal ⎭
Inability to micturate lying down	Nursing assistance to enable more upright posture
Benign enlargement of prostate	Transurethral resection

Drugs

- α-adrenoceptor antagonists:
    indoramin 20 mg nocte–b.d. (maximum daily dose 100 mg); most
        common adverse effect is dose-related sedation
    prazosin 0.5–1 mg b.d.–t.d.s.
    tamsulosin 400 mcg o.d.
    terazosin 1–10 mg nocte

- cholinergic drugs:
    bethanechol 10–30 mg b.d.
    may be used in conjunction with an α-adrenoceptor antagonist

- anticholinesterase:
    distigmine 5 mg o.d.–b.d.
    pyridostigmine 60–120 mg up to q4h.

Prazosin, tamsulosin and terazosin may all cause severe hypotension initially, particularly in patients receiving diuretics. The first dose is taken after going to bed at night. Pre-existing antihypertensive medication will need to be reduced. The only advantage in using prazosin is its cost; this has to be set against ease of compliance with tamsulosin and terazosin. Indoramin is probably the safest for use in debilitated patients.

Catheter

Discoloured urine

There are many causes of discoloured urine. The patient and his family fear that it is evidence of further deterioration. If the urine is red, it is assumed to be haematuria. The following list includes the common causes of discolouration.

Diet

- rhubarb → *red*

- beetroot → *red.*

Drugs

- doxorubicin → *red*

- danthron (in co-danthramer and co-danthrusate) → *red/green/blue*

- nefopam → *pink*

- phenolphthalein → *pink* (in alkaline urine); present in several proprietary laxatives (e.g. Agarol)
- phenazopyridine → *yellow/orange*
- methylene blue → *blue*; present in certain proprietary urinary antiseptic mixtures, e.g. Urised in the USA.

Infection

- *Pseudomonas aeruginosa* (pyocyanin) → *blue* (in alkaline urine).

References

1   Bateman DN (1994) Tiaprofenic acid and cystitis. *British Medical Journal*. **309**: 552–553.
2   Mayall FG *et al.* (1994) Cystitis and ureteric obstruction in patients taking tiaprofenic acid. *British Medical Journal*. **309**: 599.
3   Avorn J *et al.* (1994) Reduction of bacteriuria and pyuria after ingestion of cranberry juice. *Journal of the American Medical Association*. **271**: 751–754.
4   Robinson TG and Castleden CM (1994) Drugs in focus: 11. Oxybutynin hydrochloride. *Prescribers' Journal*. **34**: 27–30.
5   Matthiesen TB *et al.* (1994) A dose titration and an open 6-week efficacy and safety study of desmopressin tablets in the management of nocturnal enuresis. *Journal of Urology*. **151**: 460–463.

10 Haematological symptoms

Surface bleeding · Nosebleeds · Haemoptysis
Rectal and vaginal haemorrhage
Haematuria · Severe haemorrhage
Disseminated intravascular coagulation
Venous thrombosis

Bleeding of some kind occurs in < 20% of patients with advanced cancer. It contributes significantly to the patient's death in about 5%. External catastrophic bleeding is less common than internal occult bleeding.

Surface bleeding

Surface bleeding may be exacerbated by the effect of a NSAID, e.g. aspirin, flurbiprofen, ibuprofen, naproxen, on platelet function. If this is the case, change to a nonacetylated salicylate, a preferential COX-2 inhibitor or paracetamol (see p.27). Other options comprise

- physical measures

- haemostatic drugs

- radiotherapy (Box 10.A).

Nosebleeds

Most nosebleeds are venous. From the nasal septum (Little's area) they can often be stopped by direct pressure, i.e. by pinching the nostrils for 10–15 min. If this does not work, silver nitrate cautery is often effective. If not, the nostril can be packed for 2 days with ribbon gauze soaked in epinephrine (1 in 1000) 1 mg in 1 ml.

If bleeding continues into the nasopharynx, the source is more posterior and may require referral to an ENT department for

- balloon catheter or

Box 10.A Management of surface bleeding

Physical

* gauze applied with pressure for 10 min soaked in:
  epinephrine (1 in 1000) 1 mg in 1 ml *or* } use standard ampoules
  tranexamic acid 500 mg in 5 ml

* silver nitrate sticks can be applied to bleeding points in the nose and mouth, and on skin nodules and fungating tumours

* haemostatic dressings, i.e. calcium alginate (Kaltostat, Sorbsan)

* diathermy

* cryotherapy

* LASER.

Drugs

Topical
* sucralfate paste (2 g in 5 ml KY jelly) prepared by crushing two 1 g tablets or by the pharmacy[1]

* sucralfate suspension (2 g in 10 ml) can be used b.d. in the mouth and PR[2]

* 0.5% alum solution (*see* p.237).

Systemic
* antifibrinolytic drug, e.g. tranexamic acid 1.5 g stat and 1 g t.d.s. reduces oozing from capillaries by inhibiting fibrinolysis; either continue indefinitely, e.g. 500 mg t.d.s., or discontinue 1 week after cessation of bleeding and restart if bleeding recurs[3]

* haemostatic drug, e.g. ethamsylate 500 mg q.d.s. restores platelet adhesiveness.

Radiotherapy

Both external beam radiotherapy and brachytherapy are used to control haemorrhage from ulcerated cancers in many parts of the body:

skin	bladder
lungs	uterus
oesophagus	vagina
rectum	

- packing with gauze impregnated with bismuth iodoform paraffin paste (BIPP) for 3 days *or*
- cauterization under local anaesthetic.

Consider checking the haemoglobin after heavy bleeding. A platelet transfusion is occasionally indicated, particularly in leukaemia.

Haemoptysis

Causes

In cancer, haemoptysis may occur with

- chest infection (acute and chronic)
- tumour progression in lungs (primary or secondary)
- pulmonary embolus.

Pattern recognition generally indicates the most likely cause, e.g. infection if associated with purulent sputum or a pulmonary embolus if there is pleuritic pain.

Expectorated blood which is coughed up may not originate from the lungs. Particularly in patients with a bleeding tendency or thrombocytopenia, the bleeding may be from the nose or pharynx. Fresh blood can be from these structures or the lungs; dark blood is more likely to be from the lungs.

Management

General

- validate the patient's concern, i.e. never say, 'Don't worry about it' but, 'I'm glad you mentioned it' etc.
- re-assure the patient that, although it is a nuisance and unpleasant, life-threatening haemoptysis is rare.

Specific

- corticosteroids often stop or reduce mild persistent haemoptysis (blood-streaked sputum) associated with tumour progression:
    dexamethasone 2–4 mg o.d. *or*
    prednisolone 15–30 mg o.d.

- nebulized epinephrine (1 in 1000) 1 mg in 1 ml diluted to 5 ml in saline can be used up to q.d.s. as a short term emergency measure

- antifibrinolytic drug, e.g. tranexamic acid 1.5 g stat and 1 g t.d.s.

- haemostatic drug, e.g. ethamsylate 500 mg q.d.s.

- radiotherapy should be considered if the haemoptysis does not settle spontaneously and fails to respond to tranexamic acid or ethamsylate. External beam radiotherapy has a response rate of over 80% for primary lung cancers:
  10 Gy single treatment
  17 Gy in 2 fractions 1 week apart
  20 Gy in 5 daily fractions

- endobronchial radiation (brachytherapy) is an alternative to external beam

- cryotherapy

- LASER therapy is also useful and can be repeated indefinitely.

Gross haemoptysis

Life-threatening haemoptysis accounts for about 1% of cases of haemoptysis.[4] Many are associated with chronic or acute-on-chronic infection rather than cancer.

Haemoptysis need not be massive to cause respiratory embarrassment. When death results, it is generally caused by asphyxiation and not exsanguination. Haemoptysis of 400 ml within 3 h or 600 ml within 24 h has a mortality of about 75%.[5]

Gross haemoptysis should be treated as an emergency but conventional life-saving interventions, i.e. bronchoscopy, intubation and bronchial artery embolization, are almost never indicated in palliative care. Generally there have been several warning haemorrhages which will have prompted team discussion and a decision that the patient is 'not to be resuscitated'. The family and patient should be brought into the discussions in an appropriate way.

Adequate maintenance of the airway is essential. Lying on the bleeding side, if identified, reduces the impact on the other lung. When the site of bleeding is unknown, the patient may benefit from being placed in a head down position with oxygen and suctioning as needed. Some patients feel safer sitting upright in a comfortable highbacked chair with the head supported, tilted forward with chin down.[6] Others feel safer reclining in bed with the head and neck well supported.

Tilting the head backwards because of boredom or exasperation may restart the bleeding. On the other hand, standing up after 1–2 h, bending forward and taking deep breaths helps to dislodge clots by coughing and reduces wheezing.

If life-threatening haemoptysis seems likely, it may be sensible to have a syringe containing diamorphine/morphine and one containing midazolam 10 mg drawn up and kept in a convenient safe place, or to have ampoules readily available (*see* p.342). The dose of the opioid will depend on whether the patient is already receiving diamorphine/morphine regularly. If not, 10 mg will be appropriate; otherwise use the equivalent of a q4h dose. The aim is to reduce fear, not necessarily to render the patient unconscious. If the patient is shocked and peripherally vasoconstricted, medication can be given IV (if a doctor is available), IM or PR.

A fall in blood pressure helps bleeding to stop but a subsequent rise could lead to renewed bleeding. It is important that the patient is not left alone until the situation has resolved one way or the other.

Rectal and vaginal haemorrhage

Haemorrhage from the rectum or vagina in advanced cancer is generally associated with local tumour or radiotherapy.

Bloody diarrhoea is a complication of intrapelvic radiotherapy, e.g. for cancers of the cervix uteri and prostate. It is caused by acute inflammatory damage to the mucosa of the rectum and sigmoid colon and is self-limiting. If particularly troublesome, it can be treated with retention enemas of

- prednisolone 20 mg in 100 ml (Predsol retention enema) o.d.–b.d. *or*
- prednisolone 5 mg + sucralfate 3 g in 15 ml b.d. (made up by the local pharmacy).

Bleeding associated with chronic ischaemic radiation proctocolitis does *not* benefit from prednisolone but generally responds to

- tranexamic acid PO
- ethamsylate PO
- sucralfate suspension PR (*see* Box 10.A).

When sucralfate suspension is used for chronic radiation proctocolitis, bleeding stops in 1–2 weeks. Treatment should be continued for another week after which it can be stopped.

With bleeding from a rectal or vaginal tumour, palliative radiotherapy should be considered unless the patient is thought to be within 2–3 weeks of death. Otherwise use drugs as above.

Haematuria

Haematuria in advanced cancer is generally associated with urinary tract cancer, notably bladder cancer, but may be caused by chronic radiation cystitis.

In many cases it is mild and nothing need be done. If the haematuria is more marked, tranexamic acid and/or ethamsylate generally stops it (*see* Box 10.A). Occasionally, the use of alum may need to be considered

- 50 ml of 0.5% alum is instilled through a catheter and retained for 1 h

- frequency of administration varies from b.d. to q4h according to response

- if troublesome bleeding persists, insert a three-way catheter and irrigate with 1 l q3h–q4h.

Although the volume of irrigation may be increased to 30 l/24 h,[7] the cost of commercially prepared alum makes such an option unrealistic in the UK (£13 per 500 ml).

Sometimes a colloidal substance may be precipitated in the catheter and occasionally will block it. This is seen only at slower rates of irrigation and the problem is overcome by increasing the flow rate. Some patients develop a low grade fever and others experience suprapubic discomfort.

Alternatively, the bladder may be irrigated with cold saline 3 l/24 h. The saline is stored in a refrigerator at 4 °C before use.

Severe haemorrhage

In a patient who is close to death, it is generally appropriate to regard severe haemorrhage as a terminal event, and not to intervene with resuscitative measures.

Acute haematemesis, fresh melaena, vaginal bleeding

Acute haematemesis from a peptic ulcer or gastric cancer may be precipitated by a NSAID +/– corticosteroid.

- give midazolam 10 mg SC or diazepam 10 mg PR (if haematemesis) or PO (if melaena or vaginal bleeding)

- a nurse or doctor should stay with the patient if death seems imminent or until things have settled down

- record the pulse every 30 min to monitor patient's condition; if it is steady or decreases, this suggests that bleeding has stopped

- measurement of blood pressure is intrusive and unnecessary

- possibly take blood for grouping and cross-matching

- review need for a NSAID and/or corticosteroid

- consider prescription of misoprostol, a proton pump inhibitor, an H_2-receptor antagonist or sucralfate

- if patient survives 24 h, consider a blood transfusion (Box 10.B).

As always, prevention is better than cure (Box 10.C).

Erosion of an artery by a malignant ulcer (e.g. neck, axilla, groin)

If one or more warning haemorrhages have occurred, consider prescribing an anxiolytic prophylactically, e.g. diazepam 5–10 mg PO nocte.

Local pressure should be applied with packing. The more superficial material can be changed if it becomes saturated with blood. A green surgical towel may make the extent of blood loss less obvious and less disturbing to the patient and family. Consider midazolam 10 mg SC or diazepam 10 mg PR (rectal solution/suppository). A nurse or doctor should stay with the patient until the bleeding is under control.

Massive haemorrhage from the *carotid artery* in recurrent neck cancer is more likely after past surgery and radiotherapy and results in death in minutes; the only sensible response is to stay with the patient.

Box 10.B   Nonemergency blood transfusion in palliative care

Indications

Generally the following criteria should all be met

- symptoms attributable to anaemia, e.g. fatigue, weakness and effort dyspnoea, which:
    are troublesome to the patient
    limit routine activity
    are likely to be corrected by transfusion

- expectation that a blood transfusion will achieve a durable effect, e.g. at least 2 weeks

- patient willing to have transfusion and requisite blood tests.

Contra-indications

- no benefit from previous transfusion

- patient is moribund, i.e. the patient's condition is terminal

- if transfusion can best be described as simply prolonging a patient's death

- if the main reason is a demand by the family that 'something must be done'.

Blood transfusion helps about 75% of patients in terms of wellbeing, strength and dyspnoea.[8] Benefit occurs equally in patients with haemoglobin < 8 g/100 ml and in those with haemoglobin 8–11 g/100 ml.[8,9]

Box 10.C   Strategies to prevent NSAID-associated gastropathy

Use smallest dose of NSAID necessary.

Combine aspirin with sodium bicarbonate (short term).

Use enteric-coated aspirin.

Use a NSAID which is less likely to cause gastric injury, e.g. ibuprofen which is available without prescription because of this (see p.29).

Use a NSAID which is only poorly absorbed in the stomach, e.g. diclofenac, diflunisal, ibuprofen.

Combine administration with misoprostol.

Use a preferential COX-2 inhibitor, e.g. meloxicam, nimesulide.

Prescribe paracetamol instead of a NSAID.

Disseminated intravascular coagulation

Disseminated intravascular coagulation (DIC) is a syndrome in which the manifestations are a consequence of thrombin formation. Thrombin catalyses the activation and consumption of fibrinogen and other coagulant proteins. The resulting fibrin thrombi consume platelets. Manifestations vary from thrombotic to haemorrhagic, depending on the extent and site of thrombus formation and secondary thrombocytopenia.[10,11]

Causes

DIC occurs in several different circumstances, including

- parturition
- intra-uterine death
- after surgery
- infection
- paraneoplastic syndrome, particularly in leukaemias and lymphomas.

The common factors appear to be endothelial cell alteration and tissue injury. Tissue injury occurs in malignant disease as a result of the production of procoagulant material, such as tissue factor, being expressed on circulating tumour cells or on the vessel surface.

Clinical features

Acute severe DIC

Acute severe DIC is rare in cancer. The clinical features of acute DIC are a mixture of the manifestations of abnormal thrombosis and abnormal bleeding. In practice it is generally the haemorrhagic features which alert the doctor to the possibility of DIC. In the skin, microvascular thromboses of endarterioles and associated haemorrhage result in

- petechiae
- purpura
- spreading haematomas
- haemorrhagic bullae

- cyanosis of the extremities
- gangrene in areas of end circulation:
    digits
    nose
    ear lobes.

Areas of trauma tend to bleed because even small wounds cannot display normal haemostasis if there are profound deficiencies of coagulation factors and secondary concurrent activation of fibrinolytic pathways. The following are therefore all common

- oozing from venepuncture sites
- surgical wound bleeding
- haematuria in catheterized patients
- gastro-intestinal blood loss
- blood-stained secretions from endotracheal tubes.

Hypotension may also occur as a result of bradykinin release secondary to activation of the kallikrein-kinin system. This is seen in about 50% of the patients with acute DIC. Poor tissue perfusion and acidosis prolong the hypotension.

Chronic DIC

Although many patients with disseminated cancer have laboratory findings of DIC, most remain asymptomatic. Clinical manifestations are usually thrombotic. A significant haemostatic stress such as surgery or an invasive procedure, however, may result in abnormal bleeding.

Thrombotic manifestations include

- deep venous thromboses
- pulmonary embolism
- migratory thrombophlebitis (Trousseau's syndrome)
- microvascular thrombi with micro-angiopathic haemolytic anaemia
- IV access catheter thrombosis.

Migratory thrombophlebitis occurs more often in cancers of

- lung (adenocarcinoma)
- pancreas

- stomach
- colon.

It is less common in cancers of

- breast
- ovary
- kidney
- gallbladder.

The most commonly clinically affected organs are

- lungs
- kidneys
- CNS.

DIC can lead to adult respiratory distress syndrome, which is a common terminal event. At autopsy, microthrombi are generally found in most organs including the heart, pancreas, adrenals and testes.

Diagnosis

Particularly in the early phase of DIC, coagulation tests may be normal or not markedly abnormal. Treatment may have to be based on clinical suspicion. Repeating coagulation tests after several hours may demonstrate significant changes.

DIC is highly probable when the following features co-exist

- thrombocytopenia (platelet count < 150 000 × 10⁹/l in 95% of cases)
- decreased plasma fibrinogen concentration
- elevated plasma D-dimer concentration – a fibrin degradation product (85% of cases; Figure 10.1)
- prolonged prothrombin time and/or partial thromboplastin time.[12]

A normal plasma fibrinogen concentration (200–250 mg/100 ml) is also suspicious because fibrinogen levels are generally raised in cancer (e.g. 450–500 mg/100 ml) unless there is extensive hepatic disease. Infection and

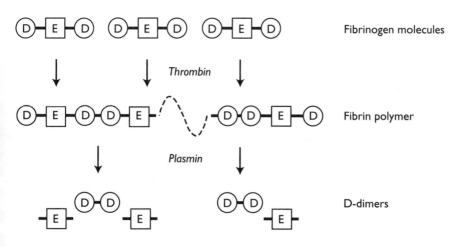

Figure 10.1   D-dimer concentrations and disseminated intravascular coagulation. D-dimers are created by enzymatic degradation of 'cross-linked' fibrin polymers. Unless fibrin polymers are being formed, D-dimer concentrations cannot be elevated. D and E are the designated nomenclature for the main domains of the fibrinogen molecule.

cancer both may be associated with an increased platelet count which likewise may mask an evolving thrombocytopenia.

Management

DIC results from a triggering mechanism activating the coagulation pathways. Treatment of the underlying disorder is curative, but this is not possible if caused by incurable cancer. If triggered by infection, however, successful antimicrobial therapy will lead to a resolution of DIC.

Chronic DIC most commonly presents as recurrent thromboses in both superficial and deep venous systems. It does not respond to warfarin. Treatment is with heparin indefinitely, e.g. standard heparin 10 000 units SC b.d. or dalteparin (a low molecular weight heparin) 200 units/kg, o.d. up to 18 000 units.

Even when haemorrhagic manifestations (e.g. ecchymoses and haematomas) are the predominant manifestations, the correct treatment is still heparin because the original trigger for DIC is clot formation. Tranexamic acid (an antifibrinolytic drug) should not be used because it would increase the risk of end-organ damage from microvascular thromboses.

Fresh frozen plasma and platelet transfusions are used to treat acute haemorrhagic manifestations.

Venous thrombosis

Evaluation and management of acute deep venous thrombosis depends on the patient's general condition and the overall aims of care. If the patient is debilitated and close to death, *no investigations are indicated and anticoagulants are contra-indicated.* If symptomatic treatment is necessary, a NSAID should be prescribed +/– bandaging +/– elevation.

For patients expected to live for 3 months or more, anticoagulants should be considered. About 50% of palliative care patients treated with warfarin have episodes of bleeding, possibly related to polypharmacy (drug interactions) and impaired liver function.[13] As a general rule, therefore, give a low molecular weight heparin as a daily SC injection for 2 weeks, e.g. dalteparin 200 units/kg up to a maximum dose of 18 000 units. Heparin is unaffected by other medication, is not metabolized by the liver and does not require monitoring.

References

1 Regnard C and Makin W (1992) Management of bleeding in advanced cancer: a flow diagram. *Palliative Medicine.* **6**: 74–78.
2 Kochhar R *et al.* (1988) Rectal sucralfate in radiation proctitis. *Lancet.* **332**: 400.
3 Dean A and Tuffin P (1997) Fibrinolytic inhibitors for cancer-associated bleeding problems. *Journal of Pain and Symptom Management.* **13**: 20–24.
4 Jones DK and Davies RJ (1990) Massive haemoptysis. *British Medical Journal.* **300**: 889–890.
5 Lyons HA (1976) Differential diagnosis of haemoptysis and its treatment. *Basics of RD.* **5**: 1.
6 Paton WDM (1990) Massive haemoptysis. *British Medical Journal.* **300**: 1270.
7 Kennedy C *et al.* (1984) Use of alum to control intractable vesical haemorrhage. *British Journal of Urology.* **56**: 673–675.
8 Gleeson C and Spencer D (1995) Blood transfusion and its benefits in palliative care. *Palliative Medicine.* **9**: 307–313.
9 Monti M *et al.* (1996) Use of red blood cell transfusions in terminally ill cancer patients admitted to a palliative care unit. *Journal of Pain and Symptom Management.* **12**: 18–22.
10 Colman RW and Rubin RN (1990) Disseminated intravascular coagulation due to malignancy. *Seminars in Oncology.* **17** (2): 172–186.

11   Baglin T (1996) Disseminated intravascular coagulation: diagnosis and treatment. *British Medical Journal.* **312**: 683–687.

12   Spero JA *et al.* (1980) Disseminated intravascular coagulation: findings in 346 patients. *Thrombosis and Haemostasis.* **43**: 28–33.

13   Johnson MJ (1997) An audit of hospice inpatients taking warfarin. *Palliative Medicine.* **11**: 72–73.

11 Skin care

Pruritus · Dry skin · Wet skin
Skin care during radiotherapy · Sweating
Stomas · Fistulas · Fungating cancer
Decubitus ulcers

Pruritus

Definition

Pruritus is an unpleasant sensation in the skin which provokes an urge to scratch (synonym: itch).

Pathogenesis

Pruritus shares neural receptors and pathways with pain. The spatial and temporal pattern of neural excitation determines the perceived sensation.

Pruritus is also characterized by its own precipitants, potentiators and blockers (Table 11.1). Histamine precipitates pruritus in urticaria by a direct effect on cutaneous nerves. Both H_1- and H_2-receptors are involved. PGs potentiate pruritus caused by other factors but are not in themselves pruritogenic.

Dry skin is a common precipitant of pruritus in advanced cancer (see p.251). Pruritus in renal failure is more complex. It is associated with an increase in dermal mast cells and divalent ions (magnesium and calcium). In patients with

Table 11.1 Factors which increase pruritus

Anxiety
Boredom
Dehydration → dry skin
Heat → vasodilatation
Proximity to another pruritic area

hypercalcaemia associated with secondary hyperparathyroidism, correction of hypercalcaemia leads to the rapid relief of pruritus. In other circumstances hypercalcaemia is not associated with pruritus.

5HT is also involved, as evidenced by the response to $5HT_3$ antagonists in pruritus associated with cholestasis and renal failure.[1] Benefit in cholestatic pruritus from naltrexone, an oral opioid antagonist, points to involvement of opioidergic mechanisms.[2] This is not too surprising given the propensity of opioids to cause pruritus, particularly when given spinally.

Causes

Genetic tendency

About 10% of the population have dermographia, i.e. an exaggerated 'weal and flare' response to a firm linear stroke across the skin. Such people are more likely to develop a vicious circle of pruritus → scratching → more pruritus → more scratching.

Disorder of skin hydration

- dry flaky skin (xerosis)

- wet macerated skin.

Primary skin disease

- scabies

- pediculosis (lice)

- allergic contact dermatitis (Table 11.2)

Table 11.2   Common skin allergens to which palliative care patients are exposed

Cream, soap etc. containing perfume
Neomycin preparations, e.g. Cicatrin, Graneodin, Tribiotic
Antihistamine creams
Local anaesthetic creams (but not lidocaine)
Alcohol (in topical antipruritics and alcohol wipes)
Wool wax alcohols (in lanolin)
Rubber, e.g. undersheets, pillow coverings

- atopic dermatitis
- urticaria
- bullous pemphigoid
- dermatitis herpetiformis.

Endogenous

- drug reaction
- cholestatic jaundice
- renal failure
- paraneoplastic, particularly in Hodgkin's lymphoma (15%)
- cutaneous metastatic infiltration
- haematological:
  iron deficiency
  primary polycythaemia (30–50%)
  mast cell disease
- endocrine:
  thyroid disorders
  hyperparathyroidism
  diabetes (usually localized and related to candidiasis)
- psychiatric.

Management

Virtually all patients with advanced cancer and pruritus have a dry skin, even when there is a definite endogenous cause. Measures to correct skin dryness should precede, or go hand in hand with, specific measures. Provided attention is given to skin care, pruritus is not difficult to relieve except in some patients with lymphoma or renal failure.

Optimal skin hydration

- dry skin (*see* p.251)
- wet skin (*see* p.252).

General measures

- discourage scratching; keep nails cut short; allow gentle rubbing
- discontinue use of soap
- use emulsifying ointment or aqueous cream as a soap substitute, or add Oilatum to bath water
- avoid hot baths
- dry skin gently by patting with soft towel
- avoid overheating and sweating; this can be a particular problem at night if a winter duvet is used in the summer or with nocturnal central heating.

Topical measures for worst affected areas

- aqueous cream (+/– 1% menthol) applied to skin after a bath and each evening
- crotamiton (Eurax) cream b.d.–t.d.s. has both mild antipruritic and antiscabetic properties; it is not often necessary
- oily calamine lotion as required (contains 0.5% phenol as an antipruritic)
- clioquinol-hydrocortisone cream (or plain 1% hydrocortisone cream) if inflamed b.d.-t.d.s.

Discourage the topical use of antihistamine creams because prolonged use may lead to contact dermatitis. If one is being used and the skin becomes inflamed, substitute 1% hydrocortisone cream until the inflammation has settled.

Systemic drugs

- review medication:
    is the pruritus associated with a drug-induced rash? (Table 11.3)
    has an opioid been recently prescribed? On rare occasions this causes pruritus secondary to intradermal histamine release
    intrathecal opioids may cause pruritus particularly in patients not previously exposed to opioids (morphine > hydromorphone); less likely in cancer patients previously receiving morphine PO or SC

- prescribe an antihistamine (H_1-receptor antagonist):
    chlorphenamine 4 mg t.d.s.–12 mg q.d.s.; particularly useful for rapid dose escalation to determine whether an antihistamine will be of benefit
    promethazine 25–50 mg b.d.

Table 11.3   Common cutaneous drug reactions

Morbilliform drug reactions	*Toxic epidermal necrolysis*
Cephalosporins	Allopurinol
Penicillins	Penicillins
Phenytoin	Phenylbutazone
Sulphonamides	Sulphonamides
Urticaria-like reactions	*Pseudolymphoma*
Cephalosporins	Phenytoin
Opioids	
Penicillins	
Radio-opaque dyes	
Sulphonamides	

alimemazine 5–10 mg b.d.–t.d.s.; 10–30 mg nocte
hydroxyzine 10–25 mg b.d.–t.d.s.; 25–100 mg nocte
cetirizine 5 mg b.d. or 10 mg o.d.; a nonsedative antihistamine useful
for maintenance treatment.

Most patients with advanced cancer and pruritus never need an antihistamine
if appropriate skin care is undertaken. *An antihistamine without skin care is
of little benefit.*

* an H_2-receptor antagonist is sometimes helpful, e.g. cimetidine 400–
  1200 mg/24 h +/– an antihistamine;[3] not of benefit in cholestasis and
  renal failure

* consider a systemic corticosteroid if the skin is inflamed but not infected
  as a result of scratching, e.g. dexamethasone 2–4 mg o.d. or prednisolone
  10–20 mg o.d.

* prescribe a NSAID in en cuirass breast cancer associated with local pruritus;
  this reduces the production of tumour-related PGs which sensitize nerve
  endings to pruritogenic substances.

Cholestatic pruritus

Pruritus associated with obstructive jaundice will clear if the jaundice is relieved by inserting a plastic stent into the common bile duct. This is done in
conjunction with endoscopic retrograde cholangiopancreatography (ERCP).
If this is not possible, alternative measures are necessary because, although

still important, skin care alone generally does not relieve cholestatic pruritus. Consider

- an androgen, e.g. stanozolol 5–10 mg PO o.d. or methyltestosterone 25 mg SL b.d.:
  takes 5–7 days to achieve maximum effect
  mode of action unknown
  may increase jaundice but this is not a problem
  masculinization generally not a problem
- rifampicin 150 mg b.d.[4]
- ondansetron 4 mg PO b.d. relieves cholestatic pruritus in 5–6 h,[5] and in 30 min if 8 mg is given IV; it is expensive
- naltrexone, an oral opioid antagonist, is used at some centres. It reduces the intensity of pruritus but generally does not completely relieve it; it is expensive[2]
- if all else fails consider levomepromazine 12.5 mg SC; if beneficial convert to 12.5–25 mg PO nocte.[6]

Cholestyramine (an anion exchange resin which binds bile acids) is *not* recommended. It is generally not effective, often causes diarrhoea and is unpalatable.

Dry skin

Description

Rough, scaly skin – either fine or coarse (synonym: xerosis).

Pathogenesis

Dry skin is an important factor in most cases of pruritus in advanced cancer, except in those characterized by wet, macerated skin and secondary infection. The most superficial layer of the skin (stratum corneum or keratin layer) needs to be hydrated in order to function as a protective layer. Water is held in the layer of oil secreted onto the surface by sebaceous glands. Dried out keratin contracts and splits, exposing the dermis and forming fine scales which flake off. The exposed dermis becomes inflamed and itchy. Scratching increases inflammation and a vicious circle is created. This is broken by adding moisture and retaining it in a lubricant, thereby enabling the keratin layer to reconstitute.

Management

General considerations

Attention must be paid to the type of lubricant applied to the skin. The greater the concentration of oil the more wetting power a lubricant has. The following is a list of lubricants in decreasing concentrations of oil

- grease (yellow soft paraffin/petroleum jelly/petrolatum)
- ointment
- cream (suspension of water in oil)
- lotion (suspension of oil in water).

Specific measures

- stop using soap
- substitute a nondetergent cleaning ointment, e.g. emulsifying wax 4 parts, white soft paraffin 1 part
- add emollient to bath water, e.g. Oilatum, Alpha Keri, Aveeno; preferred by patients and nurses
- apply emollient cream to skin after bath and at bedtime, e.g. aqueous cream BP (emulsifying ointment 30%, phenoxyethanol 1% in water)
- Diprobase (a paraffin-based cream supplied in a 500 g dispenser) is more convenient but more expensive than aqueous cream
- wet wrapping of localized pruritic area:
  apply emollient cream
  cover with wet dressing
  cover wet dressing with dry dressing.

Wet skin

Description

Maceration, blisters, exudate, pus from secondary infection.

Pathogenesis

The skin is never away from excess water. Keratin absorbs water, swells and becomes macerated → permanent damage. Protective barrier broken →

infection; usually with yeasts, less commonly with staphylococcus and streptococcus → inflammation and pruritus.

Frequent sites are those where two layers of skin are apposed

- perineum ⎫
- between buttocks ⎬ particularly in incontinent bedbound patients
- groins ⎭
- under pendulous breasts
- between fingers, particularly if arthritic
- between toes
- around ulcers
- around stomas.

Management

- dry excess moisture:
    surgical spirit
    hair dryer on cool setting
    apply an aqueous solution topically, alone or as a compress t.d.s. and allow to dry out completely
    if not infected, consider menthol 0.25–1% solution or aluminium acetate (Burow's solution)
    if infected, use an antifungal solution, e.g. clotrimazole 1%
    if very inflamed, use 1% hydrocortisone solution for 2–3 days
    generally avoid adsorbent powders, e.g. starch, talc, zinc oxide; an excess tends to form a hard abrasive coating on the skin

- protect the skin at risk with an appropriate barrier:
    zinc oxide paste where two areas of skin are apposed
    barrier cream, e.g. Drapolene (benzalkonium chloride 0.02% and cetrimide 0.2%), for legs, backs, arms, around the edges of ulcers

- monitor for allergic contact dermatitis secondary to topical agents; this may look like the initial problem.

A physical barrier is no use if the excess moisture is caused by sweating. Do not use barrier creams or ointments under breasts or in groins unless protecting the skin from the exudate from a local ulcer or urine.

Skin care during radiotherapy

Some palliative care patients have either just completed a course of radiotherapy or receive radiotherapy for symptom management as part of palliative care. In the past, overstrict advice about skin care was given to patients receiving radiotherapy. It is important not to burden patients with unnecessary restrictions while, at the same time, providing them with clear instructions (Box 11.A).

Sweating

Description

Sweat is moisture on the surface of the body which has been secreted by sweat glands in the skin (synonym: perspiration). Sweating (synonyms: diaphoresis, hyperhydrosis) is a normal part of thermoregulation and, by evaporation from the skin surface, aids cooling. Sweating also occurs in response to noxious stimuli, fear and embarrassment. In cancer patients, sweating ranges from mild to severe. Severe sweating necessitates a change of clothing or bedlinen, or both.[7]

Physiology

Two types of gland secrete moisture onto the surface of the body

- apocrine
- eccrine.

Apocrine glands develop at puberty and their ducts empty into hair follicles. They occur in the scalp, axillae, around the nipples and in the anogenital area. Secretions contain proteins and complex carbohydrates, and are under adrenergic control.[8] In contrast, the eccrine glands secrete sweat, a watery fluid containing chloride, lactic acid, fatty acids, glycoproteins, mucopolysaccharides and urea, directly onto the skin surface.

There are two functionally separate sets of eccrine glands. One set populates the entire skin apart from the palms and soles and is responsible for thermal regulation; secretion is controlled by cholinergic postganglionic sympathetic fibres. The other set is confined to the palms, soles and axillae and is controlled by adrenergic fibres. Those on the palms and soles respond mostly to emotion whereas those in the axillae respond to both heat and emotion.

Box 11.A   Skin care for radiotherapy patients (based on guidelines used by Department of Clinical Oncology, Oxford Radcliffe Hospital)

Your treatment may result in some soreness of the skin overlying the part of the body being treated. The risk of this happening should be discussed with your radiotherapy doctor and radiographer, but in most cases skin reactions are mild. Improvement occurs within 2 weeks of finishing treatment and in most cases the reaction is healed within 4 weeks.

Gently bath or shower using warm, not hot, water. Try not to spend more than 5 minutes in the bath or shower.

It is best to avoid using soap in the area being treated. The following are suitable for use elsewhere: 'simple' soap or gel; unperfumed baby soap; Wash E45.

Pat your skin dry with a soft towel – do not rub it. You may blow-dry your skin with a hairdryer on a cool setting.

Dust lightly with baby talc if you like to use powder.

Do not put anything else on the skin unless recommended by the radiotherapy staff. Certain products may irritate your skin, so please ask the staff before using anything on the treatment area.

Use an electric or battery shaver, not a razor for shaving in the treatment area.

Wear loose clothing next to the skin in the treatment area. Underclothes made from natural fibres are best, e.g. cotton.

Protect your skin from wind, sun and direct heat. You risk making the skin in the treatment area very sore if you expose it to direct sunlight, hot water bottles, electric blankets etc.

Remember

• always ask for advice if you develop a problem

• it may be necessary to change this general advice in certain situations

• if you have any questions, please ask.

These guidelines may be relaxed when the reaction is diminishing, generally about 2 weeks after finishing treatment. Continue to avoid exposure of treated skin to intense sunlight either by keeping it covered or by using a barrier cream.

Evaporation of secretions occurs constantly from the skin and the mucous membranes of the mouth and respiratory tract. The basal level of 'insensible' water loss is about 50 ml/h.[9] The maximal secretion from the 3–4 million eccrine glands in the skin is 2–3 l/h.[10]

Causes

A high ambient temperature, exercise, emotion and fever comprise the common causes of sweating. In cancer, however, some patients sweat for no apparent reason. This is a paraneoplastic phenomenon and ranges in severity from a mild nuisance to a major symptom with repeated drenching sweats, particularly during the night. Paraneoplastic sweating may or may not be associated with a remittent temperature. Several hypotheses have been adopted to explain the phenomenon

- leucocyte infiltration of the tumour and the release of pyrogens

- necrosis of the tumour and the release of pyrogens

- a substance released by the tumour which acts either directly on the hypothalamus or indirectly via endogenous pyrogen and which induces a PG cascade.[11,12]

Drugs are sometimes responsible for sweating, either ab initio or by exacerbating a concurrent cause

- ethanol (vasodilatation)

- tricyclic antidepressants (paradoxical effect)

- morphine (histamine release).

Malignant hepatomegaly and morphine in combination may represent a strong risk factor for sweating.

Sweating occurs at the menopause as a hormone deficiency phenomenon. As with hot flushes, it relates to vascular instability.[13] Sweating also occurs in men after chemical or surgical castration.

Management

Explanation

Treat reversible causes

- high ambient temperature:
    reduce heating

increase ventilation
use fan
use cotton clothing (aids surface evaporation)

- infection:
  treat with appropriate antibiotic

- hormone deficiency after castration:
  medroxyprogesterone 5–20 mg b.d.–q.d.s. ⎫
  megestrol acetate 40 mg o.d.   ⎬ effect manifests
  diethylstilbestrol   ⎭ after 2–4 weeks
  cyproterone (has weak progestogen activity)[14]

- if a tricyclic antidepressant could be a causal factor, replace with an SSRI

- if morphine could be responsible, consider changing to an alternative strong opioid (*see* p.34).

Drugs

If the sweating is associated with fever, prescribe an antipyretic (and an antibiotic if appropriate)

- paracetamol 500–1000 mg

- NSAID, e.g. ibuprofen 200–400 mg or locally preferred alternative.

Naproxen 250–500 mg b.d. may be the NSAID of choice for paraneoplastic sweating associated with a remittent temperature.[11] This view, however, has been challenged.[15] NSAIDs are probably more effective than paracetamol and corticosteroids.

If sweating is not associated with fever or fails to respond to a NSAID, one of the following drugs may prove helpful

- thioridazine 10–50 mg nocte

- propantheline 15–30 mg b.d.–t.d.s.

- propranolol 10–20 mg b.d.–t.d.s.

Thioridazine and propantheline are both anticholinergic. Thioridazine provides relief in about 90% of patients.[16]

Other measures

Although local treatment with aluminium chloride hexahydrate (axillae) and formalin or glutaraldehyde (feet) are of value in emotional sweating,[17] they are irrelevant in advanced cancer. Such treatments work by blocking or destroying sweat glands. Iontophoresis and surgical approaches (undercutting of the axillary skin, excision and sympathectomy) are also irrelevant.

Stomas

Definition

A stoma is an artificial opening on the surface of the body.

Incidence

About 5% of patients with advanced cancer.

Classification

Stomas can be classified as

- output stomas:
    colostomy after abdominoperineal resection of the rectum
    ileostomy after total colectomy or panproctocolectomy
    urostomy (ileal conduit) after cystectomy
- defunctioning stomas:
    to protect an anastomosis (temporary)
    to relieve obstruction, e.g. venting gastrostomy, tracheostomy
    to palliate symptoms, e.g. incontinence associated with a rectovaginal
        or vesicovaginal fistula
- input stomas:
    feeding gastrostomy.

Long term metabolic complications of an ileostomy, such as urolithiasis and cholelithiasis, are not seen in advanced cancer because of the short prognosis. Vitamin B12 absorption will cease if an ileostomy excludes the distal 90–120 cm of ileum.

Management

Stoma care encompasses

- rehabilitation
- skin care

- faecal consistency
- flatus.

Rehabilitation

Rehabilitation includes addressing issues such as clothing, physical activity, sexual relationships and travel. Close relatives need an opportunity to talk with nursing and/or medical staff about the stoma. This reduces misunderstandings and increases the likelihood of positive support for the patient from the family.

In the UK, a cancer patient with a stoma will receive advice and support from a trained stoma care nurse – who may well have a keen interest and/or experience in palliative care. In some oncology departments and palliative care units other nurses may also develop a special interest and expertise in stoma care.

Psychological preparation before the stoma operation is important – and perhaps the key to postoperative rehabilitation. Explanation about the use of stomas in a range of conditions helps the patient to feel less strange and less isolated from normal people. Contact with other stoma patients before and after the stoma operation is generally supportive. Several support organizations have been established in the UK, generally run by patients (or expatients) for patients, including

- British Colostomy Association
- Ileostomy Association
- National Association of Laryngectomee Clubs
- Urostomy Association.

In addition to these national organizations there are self-financing local groups or fellowships for ostomy patients in most counties and large metropolitan areas.

Skin care

Peristomal skin problems are common when liquid faeces come into direct contact with the skin. Other causal factors include

- a poorly fitting appliance
- poor skin hygiene
- gastro-intestinal upset

- abdominal radiotherapy
- perspiration
- allergies.

The incidence of serious skin problems is small with modern standards of care. A template/cutting guide should be used to help prepare the opening for the stoma in the flange of the appliance. This reduces the chance of a poorly fitting appliance and is particularly helpful if several different people are involved in the care of the stoma. All modern appliances have hydrocolloid in the flange; this helps to protect the skin.

In patients with a prognosis of several months or more, it is possible to arrange for the flanges to be precut by the manufacturers and for the patient to receive his/her own personalized supply.

Steps must be taken immediately to remedy leakage and to treat reddening or soreness of the skin. The use of wipe-on skin protection (e.g. CliniShield, Skin-Prep) is generally sufficient to allow resolution of these early skin changes. These wipes dry quickly and do not leave a greasy surface. Wipes should not be applied to excoriated skin. If necessary, a two piece appliance can be used temporarily until the skin has healed – with the flange left in place for 4–5 days before removal, thereby facilitating healing.

Orahesive protective powder (carmellose, gelatin, pectin) can be sprinkled onto raw skin. The powder adheres to the raw surface; excess powder is removed by blowing or using a fan.

Care of the peristomal skin includes the careful replacement of the appliance when it is being changed. Mild solvents (e.g. Clear Peel) reduce discomfort in patients with pain-sensitive skin, e.g. postoperatively. Warm water is used to clean the surrounding skin. The skin is dried by placing paper tissues or paper kitchen roll over the stoma and surrounding area, and pressing lightly with an open hand. Any residual mucus from the stoma should be dabbed away because if it gets under the flange of the appliance it will reduce the bonding of the adhesive to the skin.

A skin barrier (e.g. Comfeel barrier cream) may be applied sparingly if the effluent is liquid or if the appliance/flange is being changed more than once daily. It is gently rubbed in and any excess wiped off. A barrier cream is also useful around the anus in patients with a rectal discharge despite having a stoma.

Peristomal skin infection is best treated with a combination antibiotic-corticosteroid cream, e.g.

- miconazole 2% + hydrocortisone 1% (Daktacort)
- fusidic acid 2% + betamethasone 0.1% (Fucibet).

Faecal consistency

Most colostomy patients achieve normal faecal consistency spontaneously, or with the help of a hydrophilic bulking agent. With an ileostomy, normal faeces are never possible. The aim is an effluent with the consistency of soft porridge.

A high liquid output from an ileostomy leads to sodium and water depletion. This can be corrected by prescribing oral rehydration salts, e.g. Diorylate, Rehidrat. Output can be reduced with an opioid antidiarrhoeal such as loperamide (*see* p.214). Hydrophilic bulking agents are not helpful. With good control, sodium and water loss from an ileostomy is only about three times that in faeces of normal subjects. Dietary intake is more than adequate to compensate for the increased losses.

If an ostomy patient complains of continuing troublesome diarrhoea, further action is indicated

- modify medication if contributory
- identify and eliminate foods which increase stoma output from the diet (Table 11.4)
- encourage foods which are constipating (Table 11.4)
- marshmallows 5–6 b.d. will also make the faeces more solid
- if diarrhoea persists, culture effluent for possible infection.

Stomal constipation in patients with a colostomy generally relates to

- an inadequate fluid intake
- a failure to eat a moderately high residue diet
- eating too many constipating foods
- the use of analgesics and other constipating drugs.

An enema may be necessary initially, followed by the regular use of an oral laxative. If suspected, faecal impaction is diagnosed by digital examination per colostomy. A phosphate enema or an oil enema is almost always effective.

Flatus

Most modern one piece and two piece closed systems both have an inbuilt charcoal filter which absorbs flatus; most drainable systems do not. If the patient is troubled by malodourous flatus, it can generally be reduced by

Table 11.4 Foods which may affect stoma function

May increase stoma output	May decrease stoma output	May cause skin/anal irritation	May increase wind	Have been known to block stomas[a]
Fruit juices	Apple sauce	Citrus fruits and juices	Beer	Mushrooms
Beer and alcohol	Bananas	Coconut	Carbonated beverages	Sweetcorn
Caffeinated beverages	Boiled rice	Nuts	Milk and milk products	Potato skins
Chocolate	Tapioca	Oriental vegetables	Dried beans and peas	Nuts
Raw fruits	Suet pudding	Some raw fruits or vegetables, e.g. oranges, apples, coleslaw, celery, sweetcorn	Greens	Tomatoes
Beans	Cheese		Cucumber	Raw fruit skin
Greens	Peanut butter		Lentils	Celery strings
Spicy foods	White bread		Onion	
Wholemeal food	Potatoes			
Whole grain cereals	Pasta			
	Noodles			

a these foods in particular need to be chewed well.

eliminating causal foods (Table 11.4). Other options are available if dietary modification is not enough (Table 11.5).

In the UK, additives to the appliance bag are preferred to oral medication. If two puffs of Atmocol or Limone into the bag are not sufficient, they can also be used as room sprays. Limone is a more gentle counter-odour than Atmocol.

Nilodor can also be used as a counter-odour for the patient's immediate environment. A cloth or tissue with Nilodor on it can be placed nearby. Nilodor, however, is even more pungent than Atmocol.

In contrast, NaturCare is an odourless de-odorant. It works by chemically denaturing malodourous organic molecules. It can be sprayed topically around an ostomy appliance (or malodourous wound dressing) when it is being changed and onto the stoma (or wound) itself; it does not harm normal or damaged skin.

Table 11.5   Selected agents for odour control in colostomy patients (UK)

Formulation	Name
Tablets	Amplex-C (1–2 daily)
	Chlorophyll
Capsules	Peppermint (3–4 daily)
Spray	Atmocol[a]
	Limone[a]
	NaturCare
Liquid[a]	Chironair liquid
	Forest Breeze oil drops
	Nilodor
	Noroma
Powder[a]	Ostobon

a   put in the appliance bag or on a tissue inserted into the bag.

Mechanical complications

A number of mechanical complications may occur in relation to a stoma (Table 11.6). Apart from impaction, management will generally require consultation with the surgeon who fashioned the stoma. In patients with a very poor prognosis, first aid measures will generally be all that is appropriate.

Table 11.6 Mechanical complications of a stoma

Impaction	Granulation
Obstruction	Recurrent cancer
Retraction	Perforation
Prolapse	Fistula
Herniation	Necrosis
Bleeding	

Fistulas

Definition

A fistula is an abnormal communication between two hollow organs or between a hollow organ and the skin.

Causes

Most fistulas in advanced cancer develop as a result of postoperative infection and/or radiotherapy. A few are caused solely by tumour progression and necrosis.

Management

Rectovaginal and rectovesical fistulas

Management is either conservative or surgical. A colostomy, ileostomy or urinary diversion provides complete relief. On the other hand, stomas are not always troublefree. Because of this or for psychological reasons, some patients prefer not to have surgery.

Enterocutaneous fistulas

The main goals of palliative care in this situation are

- effluent collection
- skin protection
- odour control.

IV hyperalimentation may need to be considered in patients with a prognosis of more than 2–3 months. This prevents malnutrition through loss of nutrients in the effluent and promotes healing. With good supportive care, 50% of enterocutaneous fistulas close spontaneously.[18] A temporary ileostomy will facilitate closure of the fistula.

From a management perspective, enterocutaneous fistulas can be classified as

- small *or* large area (refers to surface area involved) *and*
- low *or* high output (refers to quantity of effluent).

Small area fistulas and low output fistulas (generally colocutaneous) are managed like a stoma.

Large area fistulas present a major nursing challenge because management is time-consuming. Frequent leakage may demoralize both the nurses and the patient. Advice should be sought from a stomatherapy nurse. Acknowledgement by the doctors of the difficulties faced by the patient and the nurses is supportive.

High output fistulas are generally ileocutaneous. These also present a major nursing challenge. Effluent is caustic because of the presence of proteolytic and other enzymes. Contact with the skin leads to erythema in < 1 h and excoriation in 3–4 h. The pain is often poorly responsive to morphine.

Effluent can be reduced by

- loperamide up to 30 mg/24 h; useful in low ileal fistulas because it allows more ileal absorption as a result of a prolonged transit time and a pro-absorptive effect
- hyoscine butylbromide 60–120 mg/24 h by SC infusion; reduces gastro-intestinal secretions
- octreotide 100 mcg q8h SC or 250–500 mcg/24 h by SC infusion; reduces gastro-intestinal secretions.[19]

If the fistula

- is close to a bony prominence, a two piece appliance with a hard flange is unsuitable because it will not lie over the bone; a one piece appliance is used instead

- has two surface exits, it is necessary to decide if both can be contained within one appliance or whether to use two appliances.

When the appliance is changed, help may be necessary to plug the fistula or to suction away a constant flow of effluent. The shape of the orifice is cut out of a sheet of hydrocolloid. Before applying this, any crevices can be filled in with Stomahesive paste (carmellose, gelatin, pectin, alcohol etc.) squeezed from the tube like toothpaste (Figures 11.1 and 11.2). The alcohol in the paste

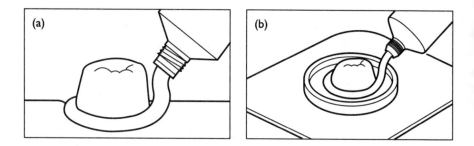

Figure 11.1   To protect the skin at the base of the stoma or edge of the fistula, Stomahesive paste may be applied (a) before or (b) after application of the Stomahesive wafer or Stomahesive flange.

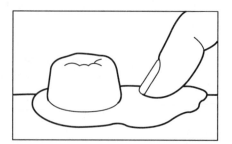

Figure 11.2   Stomahesive paste is used to fill depressions and irregular skin contours. If the paste needs to be spread more evenly, use a moistened finger or spatula. If more paste is required to form an even surface, wait 30 seconds before it is added.

will sting raw areas transiently. After applying the paste, the drainage appliance is attached. Special high output bags are available with an extension bag for night use. This enables a patient to sleep through the night without having to empty the body bag to prevent overfilling and leakage.

If the effluent is faecal there is the added problem of odour. This is embarrassing for the patient, the family and visitors, other patients and staff (*see* p.268).

Buccal fistulas

Fistulas also occur between the mouth and the face or neck. In addition to the inevitable psychological distress associated with a visible deformity, buccal fistulas cause problems with leakage of saliva and of ingested fluids. If the fistula is of small diameter, a wad of gauze changed regularly may suffice. Neonatal stoma appliances can sometimes be used and are often acceptable to the patient.

With a larger fistula, the use of silicone foam casting should be considered. Silicone foam is available as Silastic Foam Dressing. The use of plastic film results in a smoother surface to the casting. If a second casting is made, this can be inserted when the dressing is changed and the first one washed and dried. Silicone foam castings have also been used in the management of enterocutaneous fistulas.[20]

Fungating cancer

Description

A fungating cancer is a primary or secondary malignant growth in the skin which has ulcerated and which results in

- pain
- exudate
- bleeding
- infection
- malodour.

Management

Pain and bleeding

The treatment of pain and bleeding are discussed elsewhere (*see* pp 22, 232).

Exudate and infection

Measures for dealing with exudate and infection are the same as those used for decubitus ulcers (see p.273).

Malodour

Malodour is caused partly by tumour necrosis but mainly by deep anaerobic infection. Controlling malodour is sometimes the biggest challenge. Consider

- a counter-odour:
  standard household 'air freshener'
  ostomy agents (see p.263)

- a de-odorant:
  NaturCare (a chemical denaturant)
  electric de-odorizer

- metronidazole if marked malodour:
  systemically 400 mg b.d. for 10 days or indefinitely; 200 mg b.d. can
      be tried if the higher dose causes nausea
  topically 0.8% gel (more expensive)

- live yoghurt b.d.; sometimes helpful

- dressing:
  film, e.g. Opsite (totally occlusive)
  hydrocolloid, e.g. Granuflex (almost totally occlusive).

The use of oxidizing agents is less common now because of concern for surrounding healthy tissue; occasionally, however, such agents have a part to play, e.g.

- irrigation with 3% hydrogen peroxide

- packing a deep malignant ulcer with 10–20% benzoyl peroxide (Box 11.B).

Box 11.B Use of benzoyl peroxide to reduce malodour in deep malignant ulcers

---

Benzoyl peroxide is a powerful organic oxidizing agent; it often produces an irritant dermatitis and may cause a contact allergic dermatitis.

Normal skin surrounding the ulcer must be protected with petroleum jelly or zinc oxide paste.

A large cavity or an undercut margin is firmly packed with surgical gauze soaked with 10–20% benzoyl peroxide.

A dressing is cut from sterile terry towelling to fit the ulcer exactly and saturated with benzoyl peroxide; the terry towelling must not overlap normal skin.

A plastic film is placed over the dressing, e.g. Clingfilm, and allowed to adhere to the ointment or paste protecting the surrounding normal skin.

An abdominal pad dressing is taped over the plastic film with hypo-allergenic tape, e.g. Hypafix, Micropore.

Unless there is excessive exudate, the dressing need be changed only once a day.

The wound surface is cleaned with saline at each change of dressing.

Occasionally a patient complains of burning in the ulcer when the dressing is applied; this subsides within 30 min.

Decubitus ulcers

Definition

A decubitus ulcer is an ulcer of the skin +/– subcutaneous tissues caused by ischaemia secondary to extrinsic pressure and shearing forces.

Pathogenesis

Tissue ischaemia is caused by extrinsic pressure which is greater than capillary pressure i.e. > 25 mm Hg. Such pressures, possibly for periods as short as 1–2 h, may produce irreversible cellular changes which lead to cell death. This occurs particularly over bony prominences (Table 11.7). Several other factors make tissue ischaemia more likely (Table 11.8). When sitting, pressure on the skin over ischial tuberosity is about 300 mm Hg. When lying, the pressure on the heels is about 160 mm Hg on a hospital foam mattress.[21]

Table 11.7 Sites of decubitus ulcers in terminally ill patients

Major	Minor
Ear	Occipital
Thoracic spine (apex of kyphosis)	Mastoid
Sacrum	Acromion
Greater trochanter	Spine of scapula
Head of fibula	Lateral condyle of humerus
Malleolus	Ischial tuberosity

Table 11.8 Risk factors for decubitus ulcers

Intrinsic	Extrinsic
Emaciation	Pressure
Diminished mobility	Shearing forces
Tissue fragility	Trauma
Anaemia	Friction

Malnutrition, e.g.
  protein
  vitamin C
  zinc
	Crumpled bedclothes
	Restraints
	Bedrails

Dehydration	Infection
Hypotension	Poor hygiene
Poor peripheral perfusion	
Incontinence	

Neurological deficit
  sensory
  motor	

Old age	
Restlessness	
Patient moribund/obtunded	
Coma	

Prevention

There is a fundamental difference between an acutely ill patient in an intensive care unit and a terminally ill patient receiving palliative care. Although diligence must be maintained to prevent and heal decubitus ulcers, some are inevitable in terminally ill patients. Patient comfort is paramount, and there is need for flexibility rather than automatic adherence to a rigid nursing protocol.

Pressure redistribution

Mattresses vary in their pressure reducing properties (Table 11.9).

Feather pillows can reduce pressure considerably. If an airbed is not available for a high risk patient at home, consider using a camping mattress filled with water (Box 11.C). This reduces pressure more than a standard foam mattress. Alternatively, carefully laundered natural sheepskin can be used. In the UK, however, sheepskin is rarely used.

For some patients, a bed cradle to raise the bedding off the body may be helpful. Pillows can be used to help maintain a lateral position.

A pressure relieving cushion must be used for patients with decubitus ulcers who are able to sit in a chair or wheelchair, e.g.

- profiled foam (Eggcrate)

- inflatable cushion (Roho).

Table 11.9   Hospital mattresses in descending order of skin surface pressures

Type	Examples
Foam	Standard hospital mattress in UK
Profiled foam	Cyclone
Foam + fibre overlay	Spenco
Static pressure airbed	Roho, First Step
Alternating pressure airbed	Pegasus, Ripple
Low loss airbed	Kinair, Mediscus[a]
Air fluidized bed	Clinitron[a]

a   pressure less than capillary pressure – patient need not be turned.

Box 11.C   Use of a camping mattress as a water bed

Fill with water at body temperature instead of air.

When the patient lies on the mattress, top and bottom surface should not meet at any point, nor should the mattress present a hard surface because of overfilling.

The mattress is covered with a normal sheet.

The patient will maintain the water temperature. When the patient is out of bed in a temperate climate, heat is retained by an electric blanket or heating pad; the electric blanket is not used when the patient is in bed.

When filled, the camping mattress weighs about 120 kg; it can be used at home where floors are often unable to withstand the weight of a commercial water bed.

Mattresses are washed with soap and water before re-use.

Holes are mended with a bicycle puncture repair kit.

Patients should be encouraged to lift and shift their weight 3–4 times/h if their arms are strong enough to do this.

The tradition of turning very ill and unconscious patients q2h probably stems from the fact that this was the time it took the nurses to work their way round a Nightingale ward full of such patients. In modern practice, the frequency of turning depends on several factors, including

- the patient's general state of health
- discomfort when lying for long periods unmoved
- discomfort when moved
- the presence of risk factors (see Table 11.8)
- level of consciousness.

Skin care

- inspect the skin every time the patient's position is changed
- maintain optimal hygiene and hydration:
  dry skin (see p.251)
  wet skin (see p.252)

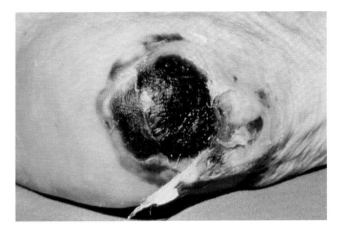

Plate 1   Black necrotic decubitus ulcer.

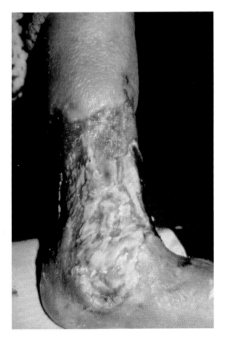

Plate 2   Yellow sloughy decubitus ulcer.

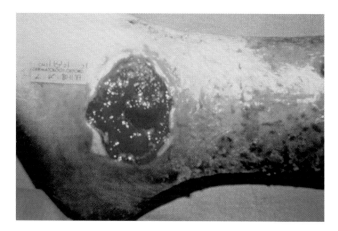

Plate 3 Deep red granulating decubitus ulcer.

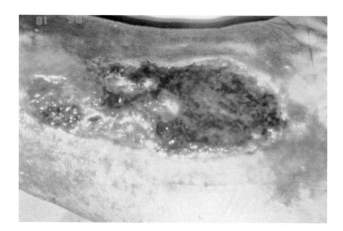

Plate 4 Superficial red epithelializing decubitus ulcer.

- avoid trauma:
    no restraints or bedrails
    patients lifted for movement and turning, not dragged
    loose clothing, smooth bedding
    avoid overheating or sweating
    use loose bandaging instead of firmly adherent tape.

Nutrition

Nutritional goals often have to be modified in the dying patient. It is not always possible to achieve the ideal of

- plasma albumin concentration > 30 g/l (3 g/100 ml)

- haemoglobin concentration > 10 g/100 ml.

Vitamin C 500–1000 mg o.d. aids healing in malnourished patients.[22] Zinc supplements help in zinc deficient patients, and may be worth checking in a patient with a prognosis of several months or more.

Management

Common conditions which delay healing are

- tissue hypoxia

- necrotic ulcer surface

- infection

- inappropriate care

- physical debility and immobilization.

An ulcer will not heal without an adequate blood supply. Local pressure must be avoided as much as possible in an established ulcer.

Growth of clean red granulation tissue can occur only after the elimination of local infection and necrotic tissue (eschar). Because it is normal for skin to be colonized with some bacteria, bacterial growth from a swab is not an indication for antibiotics unless there are clinical signs of infection. Systemic antibiotics should be used only if there is surrounding cellulitis. Systemic antibiotics may cause diarrhoea (see p.210) and encourage invasion by resistant organisms. Antiseptics are used less than in the past because they too may have adverse effects (Table 11.10). Cleanse with normal saline, or even tap water if it is safe to drink.

Table 11.10 Effects of antiseptics[21]

Name	Properties		Other characteristics
	Bactericidal (++) Bacteriostatic (+)	Fungicidal (++) Fungistatic (+)	Virucidal (++) Virustatic (+)	
Alcohols	++	++	+	Rapid onset of action at high concentrations; painful if skin broken
Phenol derivatives, e.g. hexachlorophane (Ster-Zac) chloroxylenol (Dettol)	++	++		Some absorption may occur
Iodine	++	++	++	Some iodine is absorbed; less effective in the presence of organic material; may cause contact dermatitis
Povidone-iodine	++	++	+	Some iodine is absorbed; has an inhibitory effect on wound healing
Chlorhexidene	++	+	+	
Cationic compounds, e.g. benzalkonium chloride cetrimide cetylpyridinium (Merocet)	++	++		Adsorption at the surface; weak antibacterial action against Gram-negative bacteria

continued

Table 11.10 *continued*

Name	Properties			Other characteristics
	Bactericidal (++) Bacteriostatic (+)	Fungicidal (++) Fungistatic (+)	Virucidal (++) Virustatic (+)	
Quinoline derivatives, e.g. dequalinium	+	+		
Heavy metals	+	+		Enzyme blocking; coagulatory action
Light metals	+			Astringent
Gentian violet	+	+		Strong inhibition of wound healing
Brilliant green				Strong inhibition of wound healing
Eosin				No inhibition of wound healing

Granulation tissue must be protected from prolonged cooling, drying out and trauma when the dressing is changed (Box 11.D). *Desloughing agents my cause maceration of normal skin and should be used with great care.*

For the purposes of management, decubitus ulcers and other wounds may be classified as follows

- black and necrotic – covered with a hard, dry black necrotic layer (Plate 1)
- yellow and sloughy – covered or filled with a soft yellow slough (Plate 2)
- red and clean with significant tissue loss, i.e. granulating (Plate 3)
- red and clean and superficial, i.e. epithelializing (Plate 4).

In addition, wounds may be malodorous and infected. This classification represents not only different *types* of wound, but also the various *stages* through which a single wound passes as it heals. Thus, as the condition of the wound changes, the type of dressing which is applied to it also changes (Table 11.11). The presence of infection also influences the choice of wound dressing.

Box 11.D   Commonly used wound dressings[23]

Films

Examples: Opsite, Bioclusive, Tegaderm.
Semipermeable, e.g. permeable to water vapour and oxygen.
Totally occlusive; maintain wound hydration and temperature, contain malodour.
Cannot absorb exudate.
Allow observation of the wound surface without removal.

Hydrocolloids

Examples: Granuflex, Comfeel.
Occlusive but absorb exudate, maintain wound hydration and temperature.
Facilitate autolysis of slough and eschar.
May be left in place for up to 1 week.
Also available as a paste for filling cavities.

Hydrogels

Examples: Intrasite gel, Gellperm.
High water content which helps maintain wound hydration.
Absorb large amounts of exudate.
Facilitate autolysis of slough and eschar.
Easily inserted into and removed from cavities.
Can damage healing tissue if allowed to dry out, therefore need to cover with an
    occlusive film dressing.

Alginates

Examples: Kaltostat, Sorbsan.
Highly absorbant.
Haemostatic.
Form a gel in contact with fluid, therefore easily removed.

Foams

Types: polyurethane (e.g. Lyofoam, Allevyn), silicone (e.g. Silastic).
Highly absorbant.
Good insulation.
Formulations available for deep cavities.
Silicone foam conforms to the shape of the wound surface; should not be used in
    wounds with sinuses in case debris is left after cleaning the surface.

Low adherent

Examples: Release, Mepore.
Protect wound surface.
Absorb some exudate.
If allowed to dry out, removal will cause skin damage; if wet, it is easily removed.

Table 11.11 Synopsis of wound management in palliative care

Wound type	Treatment aim	Treatment
Necrotic	Debride/remove eschar	Hydrogel *or* Hydrocolloid +/– hydrocolloid paste
Sloughy	Remove slough; provide clean base for epithelialization	Hydrogel *or* Hydrocolloid +/– hydrocolloid paste
Granulating	Promote granulation	Hydrogel *or* Hydrocolloid +/– hydrocolloid paste *or* Foam *or* Alginate sheet +/– rope
Epithelializing	Wound maturation	Hydrocolloid *or* Low-adherent dressing *or* Film
Infected	Treat infection Reduce odour	*Infection* Antibiotics metronidazole PO or topical (for anaerobes) silver sulphadiazine (for pseudomonas) *Dressing* Low adherent dressing *or* Alginate sheet +/– rope *or* Polyurethane foam *Odour control* Antibiotics (*see left*) Activated charcoal dressing

References

1   Sanger GJ and Twycross R (1996) Making sense of emesis, pruritus, 5HT and 5HT$_3$ receptor antagonists. *Progress in Palliative Care.* **4**: 7–8.
2   Jones EA and Bergasa NV (1996) Why do cholestatic patients itch? *Gut.* **38**: 644–645.
3   Davies MG et al. (1979) The efficacy of histamine antagonists as antipruritics in experimentally induced pruritus. *Archives of Dermatological Research.* **266**: 117–120.
4   Ghent CN and Carruthers SG (1988) Treatment of pruritus in primary biliary cirrhosis with rifampin. Results of a double-blind crossover randomized trial. *Gastroenterology.* **94**: 488–493.
5   Raderer M et al. (1994) Ondansetron for cholestatic jaundice due to cholestasis. *New England Journal of Medicine.* **330**: 1540.
6   Closs SP (1997) Pruritus and methotrimeprazine. Personal communication.
7   Quigley C and Baines M (1997) Descriptive epidemiology of sweating in a hospice population. *Journal of Palliative Care.* **13** (1): 22–26.
8   Kirby J (1990) Dermatology. In: P Kumar and M Clarke (eds) *Clinical Medicine.* (2nd edn) Bailliere Tindall, London. pp 1000–1001.
9   Ganong WF (1979) *Review of Medical Physiology.* (9th edn) Lange Medical Publications. pp 177–181.
10 Ryan T (1996) Diseases of the skin. In: DJ Weatherall (ed) *Oxford Textbook of Medicine.* (3rd edn) Oxford University Press, Oxford. pp 3765–3767.
11 Tsavaris N et al. (1990) A randomised trial of the effect of three non-steroidal anti-inflammatory agents in ameliorating cancer induced fever. *Journal of Internal Medicine.* **228**: 451–455.
12 Tabibzadeh S et al. (1989) Interleukin-6 immunoreactivity in human tumours. *American Journal of Pathology.* **135**: 427–433.
13 Hargrove J and Eisenberg E (1995) Menopause. *Medical Clinics of North America.* **79**: 1337–1356.
14 Miller J and Ahmann F (1992) Treatment of castration-induced menopausal symptoms with low dose diethylstilboestrol in men with advanced cancer. *Urology.* **40**: 499–502.
15 Johnson M (1996) Neoplastic fever. *Palliative Medicine.* **10**: 217–224.
16 Regnard C (1996) Use of low dose thioridazine to control sweating in advanced cancer. *Palliative Medicine.* **10**: 78–79.
17 Simpson N (1988) Treating hyperhidrosis. *British Medical Journal.* **296**: 1345.
18 Lange MP et al. (1989) Management of multiple enterocutaneous fistulas. *Heart and Lung.* **18**: 386–391.
19 Fallon MT (1994) The physiology of somatostatin and its synthetic analogue, octreotide. *European Journal of Palliative Care.* **1** (1): 20–22.
20 Streza GA et al. (1977) Management of enterocutaneous fistulas and problem stomas with silicone casting of the abdominal wall defect. *American Journal of Surgery.* **134**: 772–776.
21 Hatz RA et al. (1994) *Wound healing and wound management.* Springer-Verlag, London, p. 128.
22 Breslow R (1991) Nutritional status and dietary intake of patients with pressure ulcers: review of the research literature 1943–1989. *Decubitus.* **4**: 16–21.
23 VFM Unit (1996) *A prescriber's guide to dressings and wound management materials.* Welsh Office Health Department, Cardiff.

12   Lymphoedema

Description · Causes · Clinical features · Management
Intermittent pneumatic compression · Drugs
Transcutaneous electrical nerve stimulation (TENS)

Description

Lymphoedema is tissue swelling resulting from lymph drainage failure when capillary filtration is normal. Lymphoedema is associated with chronic inflammation and fibrosis. It can occur in any part of the body but typically affects a limb with or without adjacent trunk involvement. If left untreated, lymphoedema may become a gross and debilitating condition. Acute inflammation (whether infective or not) and trauma cause a rapid increase in swelling.

Unlike other types of oedema, lymphoedema generates changes in the skin and subcutaneous tissues, particularly when the superficial lymphatics are severely overloaded and obstructed. These changes include

* loss of elasticity and sclerosis

* increased tissue turgor

* enhanced skin creases

* hyperkeratosis

* papillomatosis.

These occur more readily in the lower limb and if there is malignant infiltration of skin lymphatics.

Although often described as 'protein-rich', the protein content of chronic lymphoedema is about 5 g/l lower than that of interstitial fluid in the contralateral normal limb.[1] Further, the protein content is relatively low in early lymphoedema (10–20 g/l) compared with long-established lymphoedema (> 30 g/l).[2] The protein content of lymphoedema is much higher, however, than the protein content of cardiac and venous oedemas (< 5 g/l and 5–10 g/l respectively).[2] Stagnant protein in lymphoedema stimulates fibrosis.

Causes

Lymphoedema may be

- primary, e.g. congenital, hereditary (Milroy's disease), sporadic
- secondary, e.g. cancer and anticancer treatments, filariasis, trauma.

In the UK, cancer and anticancer treatments account for most cases of lymphoedema

- axillary or groin surgery
- postoperative infection
- radiotherapy
- axillary, groin or intrapelvic recurrence.

Lymphovenous stasis

Because muscle activity is essential to maintain venous and lymph return from dependent limbs, lymphatic failure is inevitable in immobile patients who sit for many hours day after day and have little or no exercise.

The extra load placed on the lymphatics as a result of venous incompetence also leads to lymphatic failure. Thus, patients with chronic venous leg ulcers and swelling have a combination of venous oedema and lymphatic failure.

Clinical features

Symptoms

- tightness
- heaviness
- discomfort or pain secondary to:
    associated venous obstruction
    myoligamentous strain caused by increased limb weight
    inflammation and infection
    brachial plexopathy

- psychological distress:
    altered body image
    problems with clothing or shoes.

Limb signs

- persistent swelling of part or whole of limb; nonpitting if there is extensive interstitial fibrosis
- failure of leg swelling to reduce significantly after overnight elevation
- distorted limb shape
- enhanced skin creases
- hyperkeratosis (causing dry skin) and papillomatosis
- recurrent acute inflammatory episodes
- Stemmer's sign (the inability to pick up a fold of skin at the base of a digit); *the absence of this sign does not necessarily exclude lymphoedema.*

Trunk signs

- if the axillary fold shows signs of oedema it means that the adjacent trunk is involved. The lymphoedema may be visible, e.g. underwear may leave deeper markings on the affected side
- a fold of skin should be pinched up simultaneously on both sides of the trunk. If lymphoedema is present, the skin is more difficult to pinch up. Radiotherapy also causes subcutaneous thickening.

Measurement

By regarding a limb as a series of cylinders, it is possible to calculate limb volume by measuring the circumference at 4 cm intervals starting at a fixed point at the wrist or ankle.[3] The volume of each 4 cm cylinder = [circumference]^2 ÷ π. By programming a computer or calculator, the limb volume can be calculated in less than 1 min.

Limb size can also be measured opto-electronically (e.g. Perometer, Volometer). This method is too expensive for most centres.

Management

Because lymphoedema cannot be cured, management focuses on maximizing improvement and long term control. The earlier treatment is started the easier it is to achieve a good result. Treatment is of three types

- standard

- intensive

- palliative.

The choice of treatment depends on

- whether there is local recurrence of cancer

- the patient's general physical condition

- the state of the swollen limb (Table 12.1).

The components of treatment comprise

- explanation

- skin care

Table 12.1   Criteria for and aims of lymphoedema management

Treatment	Indications	Aims
Standard	Uncomplicated lymphoedema	Long term control of swelling
Intensive	Complicated awkwardly shaped limb, e.g. deep skin folds digit swelling severe truck swelling	Improve skin condition Reduce limb volume Reshape limb Disrupt fibrosis Restore function and mobility Reduce truncal oedema
Palliative	Local recurrence of cancer causing or exacerbating lymphoedema	Prevent or alleviate infection pain increasing swelling lymphorrhoea Maintain function and mobility

- light massage
- compression
- exercise
- positioning.

The way in which these are incorporated differs according to treatment type (Table 12.2). Success requires the patient's full co-operation, particularly with standard treatment which is undertaken by patients mainly on their own. Patients need information about lymphoedema and encouragement to become self-sufficient in daily management. They should also know who to contact for advice if they have problems.

Skin care

In chronic lymphoedema the skin tends to become dry, warty and discoloured. A break in the skin (generally invisible) enables bacteria to gain access to an ideal growth medium – static lymph. Infection accelerates fibrosis and causes more damage to the lymphatics. Careful hygiene reduces the risk of infection. After washing, the swollen limb should be dried carefully, paying particular attention to between the digits and skin folds.

An emollient cream should be applied daily to prevent drying and cracking. Apply it at bedtime so that it is fully absorbed before compression hosiery is put on next morning. Aqueous cream made from emulsifying ointment is recommended because it is cheap but any bland hand cream or body lotion will generally be satisfactory, although it may be advisable not to use one containing lanolin because of the possibility of causing contact dermatitis. Perfumed creams or lotions should not be used because they may cause irritation.

Acute inflammatory episodes

Acute inflammatory episodes are a feature of chronic stagnant lymphoedema. A hot red tender area and a rapid increase in swelling associated with systemic symptoms such as fever, sore throat, malaise and headache suggest infection. This should be treated promptly with rest, elevation and antibiotics. Because streptococcal infections are the most common, phenoxymethyl-penicillin is the initial antibiotic of choice. Erythromycin should be used for patients who are allergic to penicillin (Figure 12.1).

Because of the tenderness associated with inflammation, patients cannot tolerate local pressure. A compression garment should not be fitted until it can be worn without discomfort.

Table 12.2 A synopsis of lymphoedema management

Modality	Standard treatment	Intensive treatment	Palliative treatment

Skin care	Wash daily
	Moisturize daily
	Advice about
	  avoiding trauma
	  preventing infection
		Wash daily
		Moisturize daily
		Multiprofessional involvement may
		  be needed, e.g.
		  dermatologist
		  podiatrist/chiropodist
		  social worker
			Wash daily
			Moisturize daily
			Advice about
			  avoiding trauma
			  preventing infection

Massage	Simple massage by the patient o.d.	Simple massage for 30 min b.d.
		  by patient, family or volunteer
		Manual lymphatic drainage (MLD)
		  is available at some centres;
		  this requires a trained therapist
			Simple massage b.d. of affected limb
			  and adjacent trunk *avoiding areas
			  affected by cancer*
			Relatives taught to massage if
			  appropriate

continued

Table 12.2 *continued*

Modality	Standard treatment	Intensive treatment	Palliative treatment
Compression	International standard graduated compression garments class 2–4 Worn during the day, removed at night Garments replaced every 3 months for arms, 4–6 months for legs Bandages are used if taut fragile skin or lymphorrhoea or chronic pain, e.g. arthritis, which makes it impossible for a patient to put on a garment	Daily bandaging of limb(s) Use of different layers Tubifast to protect the skin Digit bandage, e.g. Band, Slinky Foam padding, e.g. Dalzofam Soft padding, e.g. Cellona, Velband Use of pressure pads where appropriate Short stretch compression bandages e.g. Rosidal K, Comprilan	International standard graduation compression garments class 1–3 or Shaped Tubigrip or light support bandaging, e.g. Setopress, applied daily with soft padding
Exercise	Encourage normal use Regular gentle exercise Elevation with good support when resting	Encourage normal use Refer to physiotherapist for specific exercises Exercises to be done daily after bandaging	Encourage normal use or gentle active movements or gentle passive movements Use of broad arm sling when standing if arm flaccid Full length support of heavy limb when resting

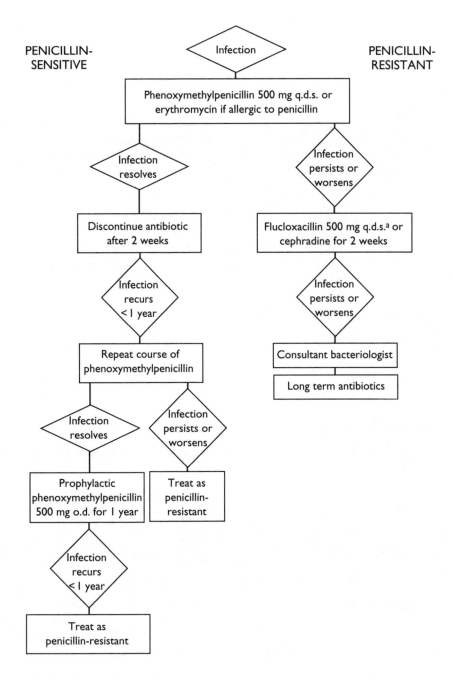

Figure 12.1   Antibiotic treatment for limb infection in obstructive lymphoedema.

a   some centres use co-amoxiclav 375 mg q8h instead. This is active against both streptococci and staphylococci but causes more rashes and diarrhoea, and is more expensive.

Fungal infections are common, e.g. tinea pedis (Athlete's foot), and should be treated with an appropriate antifungal agent. With patients who have repeated episodes of infection, long term prophylaxis is the best way of preventing recurrent attacks and minimizing fibrosis secondary to infection.

Ulceration

This occurs only if there is a combined lymphovenous disorder or if there are cutaneous tumour deposits. Because the presence of oedema delays healing, compression garments or bandages should be used together with appropriate wound dressings (*see* p.277).

Taut fragile skin

Bandaging is preferable to a compression garment when the skin is taut, shiny and fragile. Friction damage from pulling on a tightly fitting garment is avoided. Shaped Tubigrip offers a practical compromise if bandaging is not feasible.

Lymphorrhoea

Cutaneous lymph leakage generally responds to compression bandaging in 1–2 days. The bandages should be left in place around the clock but replaced if they become wet. When the leakage has resolved, compression hosiery should be fitted to prevent recurrence of the problem.

Advice to patients

- treat cuts, scratches and insect bites promptly. Clean well and apply an antiseptic cream or solution, e.g. Savlon, TCP
- take care when cutting toe or finger nails; use nail clippers rather than scissors
- dry well between fingers/toes after washing
- keep the skin supple by applying oil or bland cream
- do not allow the swollen limb to become sunburned
- use electric razors to remove unwanted hair
- avoid injections in the swollen arm, including blood sampling
- avoid blood pressure measurements on the swollen arm
- use a glove to protect the hand when washing up or when gardening etc. (upper limb)
- do not walk barefoot (lower limb).

Light massage

Massage is used to move lymph from the initial (noncontractile) lymphatics into the deeper muscular (contractile) collecting lymphatics. All lymphoedema patients benefit from massage. Massage is the only way of clearing oedema from the trunk. Clearing the trunk increases drainage from the limb.

Most women with postmastectomy lymphoedema have some evidence of swelling extending beyond the root of the arm into the trunk. *If the axillary fold shows signs of oedema it should be assumed that the trunk is involved.* Trunk oedema may also be seen in patients with lymphoedema of the legs.

Massage of the trunk and one limb takes about 20 min. Patients should be shown how to do the massage for themselves and/or with their spouse, partner or close relative. Written advice should also be given (Boxes 12.A and 12.B).

Box 12.A   Advice to patients: self-massage for arm lymphoedema

Before starting the session make sure that the area to be massaged is free of oils and creams, allowing good contact between the hand and the skin.

Lie or sit in a comfortable position.

The massage is slow and gentle with the hand moving the skin in semicircles away from the affected arm. If you just glide over the surface of the skin, you are not being firm enough; if the skin reddens, you are being too firm.

Both sides of the neck below the ears are massaged for 2 min using a slow circular motion (Figure 12.2a).

Place the hand of your unaffected arm behind your head and massage the unaffected axilla in the same way for 1 min (Figure 12.2b).

The next step is to massage the chest. This takes 5–10 min. Start close to the unaffected arm, and gently massage the chest (Figure 12.2c), progressing towards the swollen arm (Figure 12.2d). Finish by massaging over the shoulder of the affected arm.

If someone can help you, ask him/her to do the same sort of massage across the upper back starting close to the unaffected arm, moving across towards the swollen arm. This takes another 5–10 min.

Finish the session with an abdominal breathing exercise which helps to clear the deep lymphatic channels. Place both hands over the lower ribs with the fingers resting in the gap between the ribs (Figure 12.2e). Without arching the back, breathe in slowly and deeply. You should feel your fingers rise as your abdomen expands. Hold for a count of two, then breathe out slowly. Repeat the above 4 times. Relax for a few minutes before getting up.

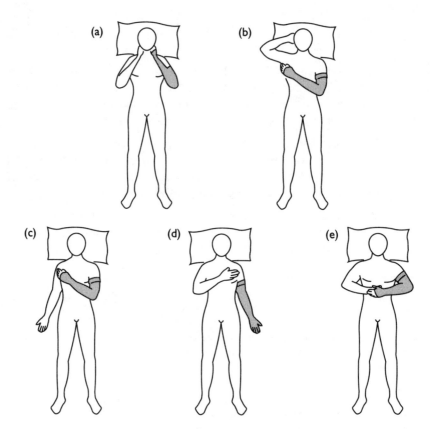

Figure 12.2 Self-massage for arm lymphoedema.

Some centres offer manual lymphatic drainage (MLD). This is a more complex form of massage which requires the services of a trained MLD therapist. It is therefore expensive and cannot be recommended routinely.

Compression

External compression is an important part of the successful management of lymphoedema. Any improvement gained by exercise or massage is lost if the patient does not wear a compression garment because fluid re-accumulates in the overstretched tissues of the swollen limb. External compression

- limits the accumulation of fluid in the limb
- encourages fluid to move towards the root of the limb
- enhances the pumping action of the muscles.

Box 12.B Advice to patients: self-massage for leg lymphoedema

---

Before starting the session make sure that the area to be massaged is free of oils and creams, allowing good contact between the hand and the skin.

Lie in a comfortable position.

The massage is slow and gentle with the hand moving the skin in semicircles away from the affected leg. If you just glide over the surface of the skin, you are not being firm enough; if the skin reddens, you are being too firm.

Both sides of the neck below the ears are massaged for 2 min using a slow circular motion (Figure 12.3a).

Place the hand of one arm behind your head and massage the axilla in the same way for 1 min. Repeat with the other arm (Figure 12.3b).

The lymph glands in the groin of the unaffected leg are then massaged for 1 min.

Massage your chest on the side of the affected leg, starting from below the collar bone and progressing down to the groin (Figure 12.3c). This takes 5–10 min. Repeat on the other side if recommended by your lymphoedema therapist.

If someone can help you, ask him/her to do the same sort of massage starting on the upper back and progressing downwards. Hand movements should be away from the legs. Repeat on the other side if recommended by your lymphoedema therapist. This takes 10–15 min.

Finish the session with an abdominal breathing exercise which helps to clear the deep lymphatic channels. Place both hands over the lower ribs with the fingers resting in the gap between the ribs (Figure 12.3d). Without arching the back, breathe in slowly and deeply. You should feel your fingers rise as your abdomen expands. Hold for a count of two then breathe out slowly. Repeat the above 4 times. Relax for a few minutes before getting up.

There are three forms of external compression

- standard using an 'off the shelf' compression garment
- intensive with multilayer short stretch compression bandaging to reshape the limb and reduce size; duration of treatment varies from 4–21 days
- palliative with light support bandaging, Shaped Tubigrip or compression garments.

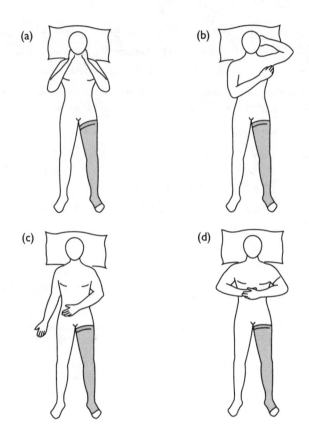

Figure 12.3   Self-massage for leg lymphoedema.

Intensive bandaging

Intensive compression is needed in about 20% of patients referred to a specialist lymphoedema clinic.

Awkwardly shaped limbs and skin folds

Compression garments do not fit comfortably on awkwardly shaped limbs, if at all. They also produce a tourniquet effect between skin folds which negates the benefit of limb compression. Padding and bandaging is used to smooth out folds and reduce limb volume before a garment is fitted.

Digit swelling

Digits must be bandaged as well as the main part of the limb, otherwise digit swelling will develop or worsen. Later, in patients with pre-existing swelling of the fingers, a compression glove should be applied with the compression garment for at least a further 4 weeks, or indefinitely if finger swelling returns after a trial without a glove at the end of this period.

Compression garments

Chronic obstructive lymphoedema needs to be treated with higher pressures than oedema associated with venous disease. If there is evidence of ischaemia, compression treatment should not be started until the local arterial system has been evaluated.

International standard compression class 3 or 4 garments are needed for patients with lymphoedema (Figure 12.4). In the UK, these can be obtained only through a hospital supplies department or specialist hospital clinic. If there is associated venous disease a class 2 garment is generally preferable. Garments provide graduated compression which is greatest distally (Figure 12.5).

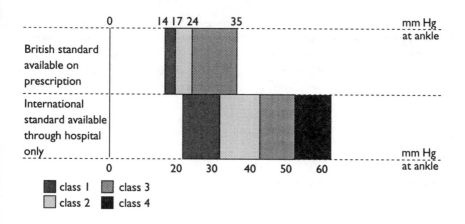

Figure 12.4   Comparison of British and International compression classes.

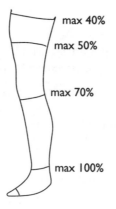

Figure 12.5   Compression profile of a stocking.

Compression garments should fit snugly around the limb to prevent

- a tourniquet effect where relatively tight
- the collection of fluid where relatively loose.

Garments are worn all day and removed at night. It is worth spending time finding a suitable garment because a patient will not wear it if it is uncomfortable.

Modern garments are lightweight, extremely strong and machine washable.
Most sleeves last 3 months; stockings 4–6 months. Garments can have their
life extended if they are allowed to 'rest' for a week every month. In this way
they regain some of their elasticity. In long term maintenance, a patient may
benefit from being supplied with two or three garments at a time.

There are some patients, e.g. the elderly or arthritic living alone, who may
have difficulty putting on a compression garment. If a friend cannot help, a
compromise may be reached using two layers of Shaped Tubigrip (not available on FP10 in the UK) or an ordinary lightweight support garment. It may
be possible to obtain help through the home care services available in the
community.

Exercise

Specific exercises have several aims

- putting joints through a full range of movements
- using arm/leg muscles to improve lymph drainage
- increasing the effect of the compression garment
- disrupting fibrosis.

A series of easily taught exercises are shown in Figures 12.6 and 12.7. External
compression must be worn during exercise to maximize benefit.

Encourage movement of the limb as much as possible because muscle contractions stimulate lymph flow by 'massaging' the overlying tissues if the patient
is wearing a compression garment. Exercise also helps to prevent stiff joints.
If active movements are impossible, passive exercises should be carried out
at least b.d.

Strenuous exercise can be harmful, however, because it induces vasodilation
and increases lymph production. Static activity, e.g. carrying a heavy object
should also be discouraged because it reduces both venous and lymphatic
return.

Place hands on top of head then slowly bring hands down to touch shoulders. Repeat x 10

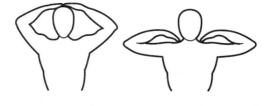

Place hands behind neck then slowly bring hands down behind the waist. Repeat x 10

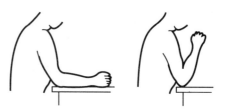

Slowly and firmly straighten arm, then bend at elbow until it will go no further. Repeat x 20

Slowly and firmly clench and unclench fingers. Repeat x 20

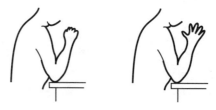

Lie flat on bed. Clasp hands together and lift arms straight up as far as they will go. Repeat x 10

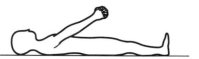

Figure 12.6 Arm exercises for patients with lymphoedema.

These exercises are best done lying on a bed or floor with the leg raised on pillows or cushions.

Slowly and firmly bring knees up to chest.

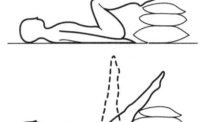

Slowly straighten legs and lower down to pillows. Repeat x 10

Slowly and firmly point foot towards floor then bring back as far as it will go. Repeat x 10

Slowly and firmly rotate feet making circular movements with pointed toes, first clockwise then anti-clockwise. Repeat x 10

Bring knees up to chest and slowly and firmly do bicycling movements (not appropriate for debilitated and older patients). Repeat x 20

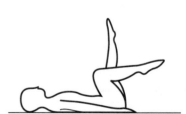

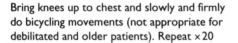

Figure 12.7   Leg exercises for patients with lymphoedema.

Positioning

Limb elevation provides little or no benefit in obstructive lymphoedema. Although it makes sense to elevate a swollen limb when resting, it is better to encourage movement rather than set aside a specific time for elevation. On the other hand, patients with leg oedema should avoid standing or sitting for long periods. Maximum benefit is achieved by elevation to the level of the heart.

Arms should not be raised above 90° because further elevation reduces the space between the clavicle and the first rib, and may increase swelling by obstructing venous return.

Avoid slings

Immobilizing a swollen arm with a sling allows fluid to pool around the elbow and can lead to fixed shoulder and elbow joints. If the weight of a grossly swollen arm causes severe shoulder and/or neck pain, or makes walking difficult, the way forward is to reduce the oedema and not to immobilize it in a sling.

If the patient's prognosis is so poor that attempts to reduce the size of the arm are inappropriate, a broad arm sling may be used when the patient is walking. It should be removed when the patient is at rest, and the arm supported on pillows preferably in an extended position. A sling is also advisable if the arm is paralysed or shoulder muscles otherwise weakened in order to prevent subluxation or dislocation of the shoulder joint.

Intermittent pneumatic compression

Pneumatic compression consists of an inflatable sleeve connected to a motor driven air pump. The limb is inserted into the sleeve which inflates and deflates cyclically.

Various makes and models are available, e.g. Centromed, Flowtron, Lymphapress, Jobst, Talley, ranging from small pumps with a single chamber sleeve to larger models with multichamber sleeves which inflate and deflate sequentially.

The small models usually operate on a predetermined inflation/deflation cycle whereas the larger models offer a selection of cycle times. The machines have a pressure dial which may range from 20 mm Hg to as high as 300 mm Hg.

The ripple effect of a multichamber sequential pump is more effective at shifting fluid than the simple squeezing effect of a single chamber pump.

Single chamber pneumatic compression has no direct effect on lymph flow; it simply forces fluid out of the limb via tissue planes and veins. The sequential action of multichamber pneumatic compression may also help to disrupt tissue fibrosis if used in lymphoedema.

If external support is not fitted between treatments, fluid will seep back into the overstretched tissues.

Compression pumps can be used for as many hours as is practical but most patients will not cope with more than 4–6 h/day.[4] Use the highest pressure that the patient finds comfortable up to 60 mm Hg. Pressures higher than this may result in the obstruction of blood flow, increased venous leakage and increased lymph production. High pressures also lead to oxygen deprivation and, if sustained, will cause nerve damage,[5,6] particularly with single chamber pumps.

Indications

A compression pump is used principally in nonobstructive leg oedemas

- lymphovenous stasis:
  immobility
  venous incompetence
- hypoproteinaemia.

Because of the likelihood of a greater impact, there is a danger of a systemic overload and heart failure. In practice this is not a problem provided treatment is limited to 30 min initially. As in lymphoedema, a support garment should be used between treatments to prevent the overstretched tissues rapidly refilling. A low pressure garment is adequate, e.g. Shaped Tubigrip or a TED stocking.

Written guidelines facilitate the optimum use of compression pumps (Box 12.C). Sometimes, treatment overnight may be the best way of achieving a good result rapidly.[7]

Contra-indications

Absolute contra-indications comprise

- extensive cutaneous metastases around upper arm and shoulder or upper thigh and groin

---

Box 12.C   Intermittent pneumatic limb compression using a multichamber sequential pump (based on guidelines used at Sir Michael Sobell House, Oxford)

Machine specifications

Centromed Macro pptt (10 chambers) sequential compression pump. Can operate three compression garments simultaneously, e.g. two stockings and one abdominal girdle
- fixed options for treatment duration: 20, 30, 60 min or continuous
- cycle time: 40, 60 or 120 sec *(normally use 60 sec)*
- pressure: variable.

General comments

Intermittent pneumatic compression is used mainly for limb swelling other than lymphoedema.

Intermittent pneumatic compression must be medically prescribed and monitored.

Explain the procedure to the patient and advise to empty bladder before starting.

During treatment the patient should wear Tubifast (cylindrical cotton bandage) or pyjama trousers or light-weight trousers.

The inflatable garments should be cleaned with soap and water between use by different patients.

External compression should be maintained between treatments during the day, using Shaped Tubigrip, TED stockings or prescribed compression garments; the foot of the bed should be elevated at night.

Circumferential limb measurements (to the nearest cm) should be made before commencing treatment and every Monday and Friday using three fixed points, e.g.
- 10 cm proximal to the base of the nail of the big toe
- 30 cm above the base of the heel (inner aspect)
- 60 cm above the base of the heel (inner aspect).

First session

Pressure 30 mm Hg for 30 min on both legs.

Use the first session to familiarize the patient with the multichamber stockings and pump, and to make sure that the treatment is not uncomfortable.

Subsequent sessions

Pressure 45–50 mm Hg for 60 min b.d. on both legs.

If the limb size does not reduce, *increase pressure to 60 mm Hg for 1–2 h t.d.s.*

Some patients may tolerate only 30 mm Hg for 30 min b.d.

If necessary, overnight use should be considered.

- trunk oedema (fluid is pushed from the limb to an already congested area)
- infection (it is too painful)
- venous thrombosis (may dislodge a recently formed thrombus; delay pneumatic compression for 6 weeks).

Relative contra-indications include

- hypotension
- cardiac failure
- renal failure.

Points to remember

- do not use pressures higher than 60 mm Hg
- fit compression garments or bandages to the limb between treatments
- delay pneumatic compression for 6 weeks after a venous thrombosis.

Drugs

Diuretics

Diuretics are of limited value in the treatment of lymphoedema unless

- the swelling has developed or deteriorated since the prescription of a NSAID or a corticosteroid
- there is a cardiac or venous component.

In patients with recurrent cancer, a trial of furosemide 20 mg daily for 5–7 days is worthwhile.

Corticosteroids

A trial of dexamethasone 4–8 mg o.d. for 1 week should be considered if tumour recurrence is the main cause of the lymphoedema. By reducing peritumour inflammation, lymphatic obstruction may be reduced. If improvement is noted, dexamethasone 2–4 mg o.d. can be continued indefinitely.

Rutosides

Rutosides (oxerutins), licensed in the UK for use in venous disease, have been shown *in vitro* and *in vivo* to have several properties of potential long term benefit in the management of lymphoedema. Capillary permeability to protein is reduced and interstitial proteolysis enhanced. Protein reduction results in less swelling and less fibrosis. In practice, however, only small returns are obtained from 1 g t.d.s. (12 tablets/24 h in the UK) when used in conjunction with the nondrug measures already recommended.[8] Under these circumstances, compliance is likely to be a problem. Rutosides are *not* used at Sobell House.

Transcutaneous electrical nerve stimulation (TENS)

Some patients with lymphoedema benefit from TENS. It has been used successfully in unilateral facial swelling associated with recurrent head and neck cancer, as well as in cases of limb swelling (Box 12.D). It is possible that TENS stimulates contraction of the collecting lymphatics and enhances the impact of the muscle pump on lymphatic flow.

Box 12.D Guidelines for TENS in lymphoedema[9]

Apply one electrode to the distal part of the swollen limb and the second proximally on to the same limb (proximal to the lymphoedema if possible).

If using dual channel TENS, electrode pairs may be crossed on the same limb, or one pair may be placed distally and the other proximally.

Machine settings
- rate: 130 Hz
- pulse width: < 130 μsec
- amplitude: start from zero and increase until the patient reports a comfortable level of tingling
- mode: start with C (conventional) and switch to M (modulated) after 5 min
- duration: start with 1 h t.d.s.

References

1 Bates DO *et al.* (1993) Change in macromolecular composition of interstitial fluid from swollen arms after breast cancer treatment, and its implications. *Clinical Science.* **86**: 737–746.
2 Crockett DJ (1956) The protein levels of oedema fluids. *Lancet.* **ii**: 1179–1182.
3 Kuhnke E (1976) Volumenbestimmung aus Umfangsmessungen. *Folia Angiologica.* **24**: 228–232.
4 Gray R (1987) Management of limb oedema in advanced cancer. *Nursing Times.* **83** (49): 39–41.
5 Rydevik B *et al.* (1981) Effects of graded compression on intraneural blood flow. *Journal of Hand Surgery.* **6**: 3–12.
6 Ogata G and Naito M (1986) Blood flow of peripheral nerve: effects of dissection, stretching and compression. *Journal of Hand Surgery.* **11**: 10–14.
7 Holt PJL and Bennett RM (1972) Pneumatic stockings to treat 'rheumatic oedema'. *Lancet.* **ii**: 688–689.
8 Taylor HM *et al.* (1993) A double-blind clinical trial of hydroxyethylrutosides in obstructive arm lymphoedema. *Phlebology.* **suppl 1**: 22–28.
9 Waller A and Caroline NL (1996) *Handbook of Palliative Care in Cancer.* Butterworth-Heinemann, Oxford. p. 95.

13 Therapeutic emergencies

General · Choking · Acute tracheal compression
Psychiatric emergencies · Pain emergencies
Anaphylaxis

General

A sense of urgency is always important in symptom management. This is helped
by setting goals and by regular reviews at appropriate intervals. There are
several circumstances, however, when one is faced with a *therapeutic emergency*
which demands an even greater sense of urgency and speed of action. These
include

- severe haemorrhage (*see* p.237)

- choking

- acute tracheal compression

- spinal cord compression (*see* p.120)

- multifocal myoclonus in the moribund (*see* p.128)

- grand mal convulsions (*see* p.129)

- psychiatric emergencies

- severe pain:
    biliary and ureteric colic
    intrahepatic haemorrhage
    bladder spasm
    acute vertebral collapse
    spinal instability
    fracture of long bone

- anaphylaxis.

Treatment protocols should be available for all these situations in palliative
care units.

Choking

Definition

Choking is the sudden inability to breathe because of an acute obstruction of the pharynx, larynx or trachea.

Prevalence

Many specialist palliative care services regularly care for patients with motor neurone disease (MND)/amyotrophic lateral sclerosis. Severe dysphagia and dysarthria are common in advanced disease. Neuropathic dysphagia is also a problem for some cancer patients, notably those with dysfunction of the lower cranial nerves seen in association with metastases in the base of the skull.

Choking because of aspiration of food, or of saliva at night, is very distressing. Patients are extremely fearful of a recurrence. A strategy is necessary to give the patient confidence that he will not choke to death.

Prophylaxis

Explanation

- acknowledge that you can imagine how terrifying a choking attack must be
- tell the patient that there are measures which can be introduced to reduce the probability and intensity of any choking attacks
- tell the patient that when such measures are introduced patients with MND do *not* die from choking.[1]

Dietary and swallowing advice

- many speech therapists have an interest in neuromuscular dysphagia and will offer advice about swallowing techniques together with advice about communication, e.g. the head needs to be stabilized with pillows/cushions so that the chin tilts slightly down towards the chest; in this position the trachea will be closed during swallowing
- liquids may be harder for a patient to swallow than soft solids
- a dietician can offer advice about maximizing calorie intake in small volume meals

- because the oropharynx may continue to function relatively normally even when the lips and tongue are significantly affected, small amounts placed carefully with a spoon towards the back of the mouth may be swallowed more easily

- neostigmine 15 mg PO 30–45 min before meals may temporarily improve ingestion.

Drug treatment

Oral morphine should be introduced as an antitussive. Begin with a trial of morphine 5–6 mg PO nocte or b.d. and then titrate dose and frequency in the light of the initial response. Many patients need only 5–6 mg t.d.s. before meals with perhaps a larger bedtime dose; a few take it q4h. The use of oral morphine is one reason why choking becomes less rather than more of a problem for patients with MND receiving palliative care.[1]

If a patient starts to cough when drinking or eating and has difficulty in clearing matter from the trachea, hyoscine hydrobromide 0.3 mg SL is helpful.[1] It acts quickly and its main impact in this circumstance is probably as a sedative. Sublingual does not need to be literally under the tongue; placing it in a cheek or by the gums is equally satisfactory. Only about one third of patients ever need to use SL hyoscine.

For the related problem of inability to swallow oronasopharyngeal secretions, some patients benefit from low doses of a β-adrenoceptor drug, e.g. propranolol and metoprolol, in addition to an anticholinergic drug.[2]

Feeding tubes

Most patients with MND do not want their dying prolonged by artificial feeding and are relieved when a doctor sensitively confirms that a nasogastric tube will not be forced on them. A few patients, generally those with dysphagia and dysarthria but little limb disability, request and benefit from one of several forms of artificial feeding, e.g. Clinifeed tube, gastrostomy (*see* p.179).

These should be offered only after consideration of the patient's total circumstances, including his general state of health and previously expressed views about treatment.

Emergency treatment

Generally the above measures are sufficient to make coughing during eating or drinking and at night a relatively minor nuisance. It is recommended, however, that drugs for emergency use are kept in the patient's home should the patient become distressed as a result of a prolonged episode of coughing, i.e. ampoules of

- diamorphine 5 mg or morphine 10 mg

- midazolam 10 mg

- hyoscine hydrobromide 0.4–0.6 mg.

In addition, diazepam rectal solution 10 mg should be available for use if necessary by a family member before professional help arrives. In practice, these measures are rarely needed.

Acute tracheal compression

This is a rare palliative care emergency. It should be responded to in the same way as severe haemorrhage (*see* p.237) i.e.

- IV diazepam/midazolam until the patient is unconscious (5–20 mg)

- PR diazepam or IM midazolam 20 mg, if IV administration is not possible

- continuous company.

Psychiatric emergencies

Panic

Panic is a common psychiatric emergency which manifests as extreme apprehension associated with autonomic symptoms such as sweating, dizziness, palpitations and 'jelly legs'. Panic is physiologically demanding and cannot be maintained indefinitely. Panic is therefore episodic but may occur in clusters.

Panic often responds to a calming presence and to persuading the hyperventilating patient to breathe slowly. Emergency drug treatment comprises one of the following

- lorazepam 500 mcg SL/PO stat (i.e. half of a 1 mg tablet)

- diazepam 5 mg PO stat
- midazolam 2–5 mg IV stat
- propranolol 20 mg PO stat.

An antidepressant is generally the best drug for maintenance.[3] The use of drugs must be linked with psychological treatment, e.g.

- exploring possible reasons for the attacks
- relaxation techniques, including respiratory control.

In advanced cancer, panic attacks can be thought of as a temporary breakdown in the normal psychological coping mechanisms of the patient. The panic attacks may well resolve as underlying fears are expressed and adjusted to.

Acute severe agitation

As in several other situations, prophylaxis may well prevent the crisis. Anxious patients are often helped by a regular bedtime dose of diazepam 5–10 mg. If highly anxious, additional rescue doses of diazepam may also be necessary. Even so, such measures cannot always prevent an episode of overwhelming agitation.

Effective sedation is necessary for the sake of the family (at home) and the other patients (in hospital) as well as the patient.

Avoid confrontation if possible and keep calm. Consider specific causes such as

- unrelieved pain
- corticosteroids
- withdrawal of:
    sedative drugs (licit or illicit)
    alcohol
    nicotine
- major psychiatric illness.

The doctor should acknowledge and accept the patient's distress, e.g. 'I can see that you are upset' and invite the patient to return to his room and/or bed so that they can discuss things further.

An attempt should be made to help the patient to express his distress. The doctor should respond to the patient's comments but also say that he recommends some tablets or an injection to help settle things down so that the patient can rest for a few hours.

If the patient will accept a tablet, the doctor should offer one, e.g. haloperidol 5 mg or diazepam 10 mg. The choice depends on the clinical evaluation. Patients with a major psychiatric illness will generally do better with haloperidol.

If the patient is already receiving regular psychotropic medication, a higher dose may be indicated. For example, lorazepam 1 mg = diazepam 10 mg. Thus, if already receiving lorazepam 1 mg t.d.s., a stat dose of diazepam 20 mg would be indicated (see p.340).

On rare occasions it may be necessary to give the patient an injection against his wishes. Although dependent on the circumstances and previous medication, haloperidol 5–10 mg *and* midazolam 10 mg would generally be a good choice, given either SC or IM. Forcing the patient to have an injection is an assault which can be justified only on the grounds of necessity. Such an approach should normally be taken only after discussing the situation with a medical colleague and other team members. If more than 2–3 injections become necessary, consideration should be given (in the UK) to applying the provisions of the Mental Health Act 1983.

The doctor should stay until the patient begins to settle down. It may be necessary for a nurse to stay longer to discourage the patient from getting up and wandering about.

The doctor should remain easily contactable in case further measures are necessary. In any case, he should contact the ward after 1–2 h to review the situation and to decide on further medication.

Agitated terminal delirium

About 40% of elderly patients who develop delirium experience distressing hallucinations +/– nightmares, and about 50% have paranoid ideas.[4] Careful evaluation may identify a reversible cause, e.g. alcohol withdrawal (see p.113). If not, sedation is generally necessary. A neuroleptic is the drug of choice

- give haloperidol 5 mg PO/SC
- repeat after 30 min if the patient has not settled
- give a double dose after a further 30 min if necessary
- sometimes 10–20 mg PO/SC/IV is necessary
- add midazolam 10 mg SC if the patient does not settle.

Sometimes it is necessary to keep the patient asleep for 24 h and, on rare occasions, until death ensues. Prescribe

- midazolam 10–20 mg SC and haloperidol 10–20 mg SC stat *and*

- midazolam 30–60 mg/24 h and haloperidol 20–30 mg/24 h by continuous SC infusion *or*

- diazepam 20 mg PR stat and q6h–q8h.

Occasionally even larger doses are necessary, particularly in a patient previously extremely anxious or who has been using denial as a main coping mechanism. As the patient becomes less able to control his thoughts, unresolved fears break through into the now confused mind with devastating results.

If the patient fails to settle with midazolam 100 mg/24 h and haloperidol 30 mg/24 h, consider phenobarbital 200 mg SC/IM stat and 800–1600 mg/24 h by continuous SC infusion.

Some centres use chlorpromazine 50–100 mg q4h IM or levomepromazine 200–300 mg/24 h (*see* p.334). In situations where convulsions are a definite risk, i.e. patients with multifocal myoclonus or a cerebral tumour, midazolam should be prescribed as well, e.g. 30–60 mg/24 h SC.

Propofol, an ultra-fast acting anaesthetic agent, provides yet another option.[5,6] Propofol is given IV as a 1% solution (10 mg/ml) in doses ranging from 5–70 mg/h (0.5–7 ml) using a computer-controlled volumetric infusion pump. 10 mg/h (1 ml) is a typical starting dose with 10 mg/h increments every 15 min until a satisfactory level of sedation is achieved. Any change in rate has an effect in 5–10 min. If it is necessary to increase the level of sedation quickly, boluses of 20–50 mg can be given by increasing the rate to 1 ml/min for 2–5 min. If the patient is too 'deep', the infusion should be turned off for 2–3 min and then restarted at a lower rate. It is important to replenish the infusion quickly when a container empties, otherwise the sedation will wear off after a few minutes.

Pain emergencies

Biliary and ureteric colic

The treatment of choice for biliary colic is an IM or IV injection of a NSAID, e.g. diclofenac 75 mg.[7] If this fails to relieve adequately in 20–30 min, it should be supplemented by diamorphine SC/IV 5 mg or morphine SC/IV 10 mg.

Alternatively, if already receiving oral morphine for cancer pain management, give

- a double dose of morphine PO *or*

- an injection of diamorphine/morphine equal in mg to the previous regular PO dose; this will have treble/double the effect of the oral dose.

Intrahepatic haemorrhage

Occasionally a patient with marked malignant hepatomegaly experiences increasingly severe and persistent right upper quadrant pain. Unless associated features suggest an alternative diagnosis, e.g. perforated peptic ulcer or cholecystitis, the most likely diagnosis is an intrahepatic haemorrhage causing acute distension of the hepatic capsule. When this is the case

- explain the cause to the patient
- give *double* the previous oral analgesic morphine requirement *or*
- if the patient has already taken an extra rescue dose of morphine with inadequate relief, *treble* the previous oral morphine dose.

This is an acute phenomenon which resolves as the hepatic capsule adapts and the haematoma is resorbed. Therefore, advise the patient that in 6–8 days time his analgesic requirement will be the same as before the haemorrhage.

Make tentative dose reductions after 3 days, or sooner if the patient is comfortable and complaining of drowsiness. Failure to reduce the dose will result in

- unnecessary tolerance
- increased adverse effects to morphine:
    drowsiness
    nausea and vomiting
    constipation.

Bladder spasm (see p.226)

Acute vertebral collapse

Often the patient is already taking regular analgesics for bone pain and, before being seen by a doctor, will already have taken one or more rescue doses of oral morphine. If these have failed to give adequate relief, it is necessary to *treble* the previous satisfactory dose of morphine for up to several weeks.

Palliative radiotherapy is generally beneficial but it may take 4–6 weeks to achieve maximal relief. In patients with troublesome secondary muscle spasm, diazepam 5 mg stat and 5–10 mg nocte may help.

For those with associated troublesome nerve compression pain, dexamethasone 4–8 mg o.d. may also help. Alternatively, some patients benefit from epidural depot methylprednisolone 80 mg in 2 ml. This can be repeated once or twice at daily or weekly intervals.

Spinal instability

In terms of distress, spinal instability related to metastatic cancer is comparable to a pathological fracture of a long bone. Fortunately, it occurs rarely. It can cause excruciating back pain on even slight movement which overwhelms the patient. Options include

- epidural analgesia with morphine and bupivacaine
- orthopaedic surgery to stabilize the spine:[8]
    anterior spinal fusion
    posterior stabilization.

If these are not available, consider the use of nitrous oxide (50% with oxygen) before and during movement.

Pathological fracture of long bone

Consider surgery. With cancer of breast and prostate, patients often survive months or years, whereas with cancer of bronchus and melanoma, patients often die within a few weeks.

Ensure that adequate analgesics are provided together with night sedation. If surgery is planned, ensure that pre-fracture analgesics are continued and that additional as needed postoperative medication is prescribed at an appropriate dose level. This includes giving advice on the dose of SC diamorphine or morphine to replace oral morphine in the immediate postoperative period when the patient is unable to take medication by mouth.

Humerus

Often treated conservatively

- use a standard triangular sling; apart from giving physical support, it warns people to 'handle with care' *or*
- splint arm to trunk with Netelast and/or Velcro.

Femur

Generally treated surgically

- immobilize leg with pillows

- use appropriate nursing techniques for turning the patient in bed, e.g. 'logrolling'

- administer a local anaesthetic femoral nerve block with 10 ml of 0.5% bupivacaine before obtaining a radiograph

- use a Thomas splint or bandage the legs together if transferring to orthopaedic/accident service (plus local anaesthetic block)

- if treating conservatively, consider an infusion of epidural morphine and bupivacaine.

Anaphylaxis

Causes

Wasp and bee stings and certain foods, food additives and tablet excipients occasionally cause anaphylaxis. In palliative care, anaphylaxis is rare and is generally associated with drugs, e.g.

- antibiotics

- aspirin and other NSAIDs.

Anaphylaxis is specific to a given drug or chemically-related class of drugs. Anaphylaxis is more likely after parenteral administration.

Clinical features

Anaphylaxis is characterized by the following symptoms and signs which develop *within seconds or minutes* of taking the causal drug

- flushing

- palpitations

- weakness

- dizziness

- tingling of the extremities

- urticaria

- angio-oedema

- agitation.

Asthma occurs in < 10%; hypotension, pallor and other manifestations of shock are uncommon.[9] Patients with systemic lupus erythematosus or with aspirin-induced asthma are at greater risk, although only a minority of those developing anaphylaxis have a history of asthma or chronic rhinitis.

Management

Anaphylaxis requires prompt treatment with epinephrine (adrenaline) backed up by an antihistamine and hydrocortisone (Box 13.A). *Corticosteroids are only of secondary value because their impact is not immediate.*

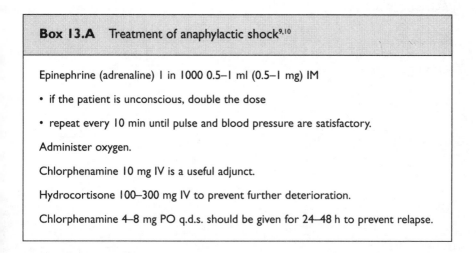

Box 13.A Treatment of anaphylactic shock[9,10]

Epinephrine (adrenaline) 1 in 1000 0.5–1 ml (0.5–1 mg) IM

• if the patient is unconscious, double the dose

• repeat every 10 min until pulse and blood pressure are satisfactory.

Administer oxygen.

Chlorphenamine 10 mg IV is a useful adjunct.

Hydrocortisone 100–300 mg IV to prevent further deterioration.

Chlorphenamine 4–8 mg PO q.d.s. should be given for 24–48 h to prevent relapse.

References

1   O'Brien T *et al.* (1992) Motor neurone disease: a hospice perspective. *British Medical Journal.* **304**: 471–473.
2   Newall AR *et al.* (1996) The control of oral secretions in bulbar ALS/MND. *Journal of Neurological Sciences.* **139** (suppl): 43–44.
3   Tyrer P (1989) Treating panic. *British Medical Journal.* **298**: 201.
4   Lipowski ZJ (1983) Transient cognitive disorders (delirium, acute confusional states) in the elderly. *American Journal of Psychiatry.* **140**: 1426–1436.
5   Moyle J (1995) The use of propofol in palliative medicine. *Journal of Pain and Symptom Management.* **10**: 643–646.

6   Mercadante S *et al.* (1995) Propofol in terminal care. *Journal of Pain and Symptom Management.* **10**: 639–642.
7   Anonymous (1987) NSAIDs for renal and biliary colic: intramuscular diclofenac. *Drug and Therapeutics Bulletin.* **25**: 85–86.
8   Fallon MT and O'Neill WM (1993) Spinal surgery in the treatment of metastatic back pain: three case reports. *Palliative Medicine.* **7**: 235–238.
9   Szczeklik A (1986) Analgesics, allergy and asthma. *Drugs.* **32** (suppl 4): 148–163.
10   *British National Formulary* (1995) A joint publication of the British Medical Association and the Royal Pharmaceutical Society of Great Britain, London. No. 29 (March): 135–137.

14   Drug profiles

Corticosteroids · Antacids · Prokinetics
Psychotropics · Neuroleptics · Haloperidol
Phenothiazines · Benzodiazepines · Diazepam
Midazolam · Antidepressants · Hyoscine
Anticholinergic effects
Drug-induced movement disorders

Corticosteroids

Corticosteroids are used for many reasons in advanced cancer (Table 14.1). Inclusion in the table does *not* mean that a corticosteroid is necessarily the treatment of choice in that situation.

At Sobell House, dexamethasone is the corticosteroid of choice. It is generally given in a single daily dose. Dexamethasone has a duration of effect of 36–54 h, compared with 18–36 h for prednisolone (Table 14.2).

Dexamethasone is 7 times more potent than prednisolone. Thus, 2 mg of dexamethasone is approximately equivalent to 15 mg of prednisolone. Dexamethasone is available in 0.5 mg and 2 mg tablets, and also as an injection. Prednisolone is available in a range of sizes from 1–25 mg.

The initial daily dose varies according to indication and fashion, ranging from dexamethasone 2–4 mg (prednisolone 15–30 mg) for anorexia to 16–32 mg for spinal cord compression. A dose of 8–16 mg is generally used for raised intracranial pressure.

Oral candidiasis and ankle oedema are common adverse effects. Moonfacing, hyperphagia, weight gain, myopathy or diabetes mellitus may necessitate dose reduction and, sometimes, cessation of treatment (Table 14.3). Agitation, insomnia or a more florid psychiatric disturbance may be precipitated by corticosteroids – either when commencing or stopping treatment.

Apart from hydrocortisone, corticosteroids should generally be given in a single daily dose in the morning to ease compliance and to prevent insomnia. Even so, temazepam or diazepam at bedtime is sometimes needed to counter insomnia or agitation.

Table 14.1 Indications for corticosteroids in advanced cancer

Specific

Spinal cord compression
Nerve compression
Dyspnoea
   pneumonitis (after radiotherapy)
   lymphangitis carcinomatosa
   tracheal compression/stridor
Superior vena caval obstruction
Pericardial effusion
Haemoptysis
Obstruction of hollow viscus
   bronchus
   ureter
   [bowel]
Hypercalcaemia (in corticosteroid-responsive tumours, *see* p.138)
Radiation-induced inflammation
Leuco-erythroblastic anaemia
Rectal discharge (give PR)
Sweating

Pain relief

Raised intracranial pressure
Nerve compression
Spinal cord compression
Metastatic arthralgia
[Bone pain]

Hormone therapy

Replacement
Anticancer

General

To improve appetite
To enhance sense of wellbeing
To improve strength

Table 14.2 Adrenal corticosteroids[1]

Drug	Anti-inflammatory potency	Equivalent dose (mg)	Sodium retaining potency	Daily dose (mg) above which hypothalamopituitary axis suppression is possible		Plasma halflife (min)	Plasma Biological halflife (h)
				Males	Females		
Hydrocortisone	1	20	++	20–30	15–25	90	8–12
Cortisone	0.8	25	++	25–35	20–30	90	8–12
Prednisone	3.5	5	+	7.5–10	7.5	⩾ 200	18–36
Prednisolone	4	5	+	7.5–10	7.5	⩾ 200	18–36
Methylprednisolone	5	4	–	7.5–10	7.5	⩾ 200	18–36
Triamcinolone	5	4	–	7.5–10	7.5	⩾ 200	18–36
Paramethasone	10	2	–	2.5–5	2.5–5	⩾ 300	36–54
Betamethasone	25–30	0.7–0.8	–	1–1.5	1–1.5	⩾ 300	36–54
Dexamethasone	25–30	0.7–0.8	–	1–1.5	1–1.5	⩾ 300	36–54

Table 14.3   Disadvantages of corticosteroids

Glucocorticosteroid effects

Diabetes
Osteoporosis
Avascular bone necrosis
Mental disturbance
   paranoid psychosis
   depression
   euphoria
Muscle wasting
Peptic ulceration (if given with a NSAID)
Infection
   septicaemia (may delay recognition)
   tuberculosis
Suppression of growth in child

Mineralocorticosteroid effects

Hypertension
Sodium and water retention
Potassium loss

Cushing's syndrome

Moonface
Striae
Acne

Steroid cataract

If prednisolone 15 mg or equivalent taken daily for several years = 75% risk

Corticosteroid myopathy

The onset of corticosteroid myopathy generally occurs in the third month of treatment with dexamethasone $\geq$ 4 mg o.d. or prednisolone $\geq$ 40 mg o.d. It can occur earlier and with lower doses (Table 14.4). An appropriate level of suspicion is the main prerequisite for diagnosis. For example, a patient may walk into the consultation room with no difficulty but subsequently have difficulty getting up from the sitting position. If the chronological sequence fits with corticosteroid myopathy, a presumptive diagnosis should be made and the following steps taken

- explanation to patient and family

Table 14.4   Corticosteroid myopathy

Symptoms

Generally insidious onset
Diffuse myalgia may occur
Difficulty with
    climbing stairs } early
    standing up
    arm elevation
    holding head up } late
    distal extremities

Signs

Weakness } usually symmetrical
Wasting
Hypercortisolism
    moonface
    abdominal striae
    ankle oedema

Normal

Reflexes
Sensation
Enzymes (AST, CPK, aldolase)

Differential diagnosis

Hypokalaemia
Hypophosphataemia
Paraneoplastic neuropathy/myopathy
Lumbosacral plexopathy
Spinal cord compression

- discuss the need to compromise between maximizing therapeutic benefit and minimizing adverse effects
- halve corticosteroid dose (generally possible as a single step)
- arrange for physiotherapy (disuse exacerbates myopathy)
- emphasize that weakness should improve after 3–4 weeks
- review after 2–3 weeks to ensure that there is no further deterioration
- consider changing from dexamethasone to prednisolone (nonfluorinated corticosteroids cause less myopathy).

Steroid pseudorheumatism

Patients receiving corticosteroids for rheumatoid arthritis occasionally develop diffuse pains, malaise and pyrexia (Table 14.5). This syndrome is called steroid pseudorheumatism. It is also sometimes seen in cancer patients receiving large doses of corticosteroids or when a very high dose is reduced rapidly to a lower maintenance level. Cancer patients most likely to be affected are those

- receiving 100 mg of prednisolone daily for several days in association with chemotherapy
- with spinal cord compression given dexamethasone 100 mg daily for several days
- on high doses of dexamethasone to reduce raised intracranial pressure associated with brain metastases
- reducing to an ordinary maintenance dose after a prolonged course.

Table 14.5   Steroid withdrawal pain or pseudorheumatism[2]

Myalgia and cramps	Malaise
Arthralgia	Pyrexia
Tendon pains	Tachycardia
Bone pains	Restlessness
Weakness	Emotional lability
Fatigue	Memory deficit

Drug interactions

Corticosteroids antagonize the effects of

- antidiabetic therapy (both oral hypoglycaemics and insulin)
- antihypertensives (because of their mineralocorticosteroid effect)
- diuretics (because of their mineralocorticosteroid effect).

There is an increased risk of hypokalaemia if high doses of corticosteroids are prescribed with

- β_2-sympathomimetics (e.g. salbutamol, terbutaline)
- carbenoxolone.

The metabolism of corticosteroids is accelerated by

- aminoglutethimide (dexamethasone only)
- anticonvulsants:
  carbamazepine
  phenobarbital
  phenytoin
  primidone
- rifampicin.

The rate of metabolism of the longer acting glucocorticosteroids, e.g. dexamethasone, is affected more than prednisolone or hydrocortisone. Thus, because phenytoin and phenobarbital can reduce the bio-availability of dexamethasone to 25–50%, the dose should be doubled (or more) if prescribed concurrently.[3]

Antacids

An antacid is a chemical substance taken by mouth to neutralize gastric acid. Generic antacids include

- sodium bicarbonate
- magnesium salts (cause diarrhoea)
- aluminium hydroxide (causes constipation)
- hydrotalcite/magnesium aluminium carbonate
- calcium carbonate.

Proprietary preparations generally contain a mixture of magnesium and aluminium so as to neutralize any effect on bowel habit. They may also contain sodium bicarbonate.

Some antacids contain significant amounts of sodium. This may be important in patients with hypertension or cardiac failure. *Liquid Gaviscon and magnesium trisilicate mixture both contain > 6 mmol/10 ml* compared with 0.1 mmol/10 ml in Asilone. Regular use of sodium bicarbonate may cause sodium loading and metabolic alkalosis.

Aluminium hydroxide binds dietary phosphate. It is of benefit in patients with hyperphosphataemia in renal failure. Long term complications of phosphate depletion and osteomalacia are not generally an issue in advanced cancer.

Hydrotalcite binds bile salts and is therefore of specific benefit in patients with bile salt reflux, e.g. after certain forms of gastroduodenal surgery.

Regular use of calcium carbonate may cause hypercalcaemia, particularly if taken with sodium bicarbonate.

Therapeutic considerations

* a 20 ml dose of most antacids q2h will reduce gastric acidity by up to 50%. H_2-receptor antagonists have a similar effect during the day but achieve greater nocturnal inhibition (2/3 compared with 1/3)

* when fasting, conventional doses act for 20–40 min

* a 20 ml dose 1 h after a meal neutralizes acid for 2 h

* antacids delay gastric emptying, except sodium bicarbonate

* some antacids contain peppermint oil which helps belching by decreasing the tone of the lower oesophageal sphincter; the mint flavour may be a limiting factor in treatment

* most tablets feel gritty when sucked; this also may be a limiting factor

* antacids containing barbiturates and/or anticholinergic agents are *not* recommended

* the cheapest preparations are:
  magnesium trisilicate BP
  aluminium hydroxide gel BP   } may be given alone or as a mixture.

Special preparations

Some antacids contain additional substances for use in specific situations

* alginic acid (in Gaviscon) prevents oesophageal reflux pain by forming an inert low density raft on the top of the acid stomach contents. Gaviscon needs both *acid* and *air bubbles* to produce the raft. It may be less effective if used with an H_2-receptor antagonist (reduces acid) and/or antiflatulent (reduces air bubbles). Liquid Gaviscon contains 6 mmol of sodium/10 ml

* dimeticone (dimethylpolysiloxane) is an antifoaming agent present in Asilone, a proprietary antacid. By facilitating belching, dimeticone eases

flatulence, distension and postprandial gastric distension pain. Dimeticone-containing antacids are as effective as Gaviscon in the treatment of acid reflux.[4] Asilone should be used in preference to Gaviscon because it is cheaper and contains almost no sodium. Asilone is also first line treatment for hiccup (see p.152)

- oxetacaine (in Mucaine) eases reflux pain by coating and anaesthetizing damaged oesophageal mucosa. Use should be limited to short term treatment of painful oesophagitis, e.g. 5–10 ml 15 min before meals and/or drinks, until specific treatment of the underlying condition (hyperacidity, candidiasis) achieves healing.

Prokinetics

Prokinetics accelerate gastro-intestinal transit by a neurohumoral mechanism. By convention, the term has been restricted to drugs which

- co-ordinate antroduodenal contractions
- accelerate gastroduodenal transit (Tables 14.6 and 14.7).

Bulk-forming agents and other laxatives are not included, despite the overlap of site of action between a panprokinetic, e.g. cisapride, and colonic stimulant laxatives, e.g. senna. Drugs which cause diarrhoea by increasing gut secretions, e.g. misoprostol, are also not included.

Some drugs increase contractile motor activity but are not consistently associated with decreased transit time because the contractility is not co-ordinated between adjacent intestinal segments, e.g. bethanechol. Such drugs are promotility but not prokinetic.

Erythromycin is the only readily available motilin agonist. Its action is mainly

Table 14.6 Gastro-intestinal prokinetics

Class	Examples	Main site of action
Dopamine type 2 antagonist	Domperidone	Stomach
	Metoclopramide	Stomach
$5HT_4$ agonist	Metoclopramide	Stomach → jejunum
	Cisapride	Stomach → colon
Motilide (motilin agonist)	Erythromycin	Stomach

Table 14.7 Effects of prokinetics on gastro-intestinal motility[5]

	Metoclopramide	Domperidone	Cisapride	Erythromycin
Increases oesophageal peristalsis	?	0	+	0
Increases lower oesophageal sphincter pressure	+	0	++	++
Enhances antral contractility and speeds gastric emptying	+	+	++	+++
Enhances gallbladder emptying	0	0[a]	++	+
Enhances small bowel transit				
after food	NK	0	++	–
fasting	+	0[a]	NK	+
Speeds colon transit	0	0	+	0

NK not known; 0 no effect; +, ++, +++ definite prokinetic effect; ? dubious effect; – antikinetic effect.

a although formal experiments have not been undertaken in relation to its impact on gallbladder function or postprandial small bowel transit, it can be predicted that domperidone will have no effect because dopamine type 2 receptors in the gastro-intestinal tract are restricted to the proximal and distal ends of the stomach, and adjacent parts of the oesophagus and duodenum.

limited to the stomach; tolerance to its effect generally develops after a few days. Dopamine type 2 antagonists block the inhibitory dopaminergic 'brake' on gastric emptying which is induced by stress, anxiety and nausea. In contrast $5HT_4$ agonists have a direct excitatory effect.

In practice, the choice of prokinetic lies between metoclopramide (dopamine antagonist and $5HT_4$ agonist), domperidone (dopamine antagonist) and cisapride ($5HT_4$ agonist). These act by triggering a cholinergic system in the gastro-intestinal wall (Figure 14.1); an action which is impeded but not blocked by opioids.

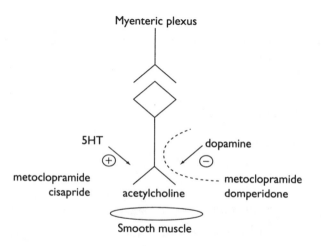

Figure 14.1 Schematic representation of drug effects on antroduodenal co-ordination via a postganglionic effect on the cholinergic nerves from the myenteric plexus.

⊕ stimulatory effect of 5HT triggered by metoclopramide and cisapride; ⊖ inhibitory effect of dopamine; - - - blockade of dopamine inhibition by metoclopramide and domperidone.

On the other hand, anticholinergics block the cholinergic receptors on the intestinal muscle fibres.[6] Thus, depending on the dose, anticholinergics will block the prokinetic effect of $5HT_4$ agonists to a greater or lesser extent. It is, therefore, pharmacological nonsense to prescribe prokinetics and anti-cholinergics concurrently. Metoclopramide and domperidone, however, will still exert an anti-emetic effect in the area postrema (Figure 14.2).

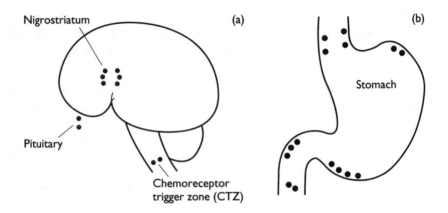

Figure 14.2 Site of dopamine receptors in (a) the brain and (b) the stomach.

Use of prokinetics in palliative care

Prokinetics are used in various conditions in palliative care (Table 14.8). Despite its dual mechanism of action, metoclopramide is not more potent than domperidone when used in standard doses, e.g. 10 mg t.d.s.–q.d.s., to treat gastro-oesophageal reflux or delayed gastric emptying. When treating functional bowel obstruction, however, metoclopramide is clearly preferable.

The prokinetic effect of cisapride is more diffuse than metoclopramide and it is some 2–4 times more potent.[7,8] It reverses opioid-induced delayed gastric

Table 14.8 Indications for prokinetics in advanced cancer

Gastro-oesophageal reflux
Gastroparesis
    dysmotility dyspepsia
    drug-induced
    paraneoplastic visceral neuropathy

Functional bowel obstruction
    duodenum (cancer of head of pancreas)
    drug-induced

Constipation (cisapride only)

Irritable bowel syndrome (cisapride only)

emptying more completely. Despite its expense, cisapride should be prescribed if symptoms of delayed gastric emptying (opioid-induced or cancer-related autonomic neuropathy) do not respond to metoclopramide. Its value in functional bowel obstruction has not been evaluated. Given a plasma halflife of 6–12 h, cisapride can generally be given 10–20 mg b.d.

Metoclopramide is the only prokinetic available as an injection (Table 14.9). High dose parenteral metoclopramide (up to 240 mg/24 h) is used at some centres in bowel obstruction. This is *not* recommended. It is acting as a 5HT$_3$ antagonist at this dose and a more specific drug should be used if needed (Table 14.10). The same holds true for chemotherapeutic vomiting.

Table 14.9   Prokinetic preparations available in the UK

Drug	Tablet/Capsule	Liquid	Suppository	Injection
Metoclopramide	10 mg	5 mg/5 ml (solution, syrup)	–	10 mg/2 ml
	15, 30 mg m/r			100 mg/20 ml
Domperidone	10 mg	5 mg/5 ml (suspension)	30 mg[a]	–
Cisapride	10 mg	5 mg/5 ml (suspension)	30 mg[b]	–

a   equivalent to 10 mg PO
b   equivalent to 13 mg PO; unlicensed in UK but can be imported from Belgium on a named-patient basis.

Table 14.10   5HT$_3$ and 5HT$_4$ modulation[5]

	5HT$_3$ antagonist	5HT$_4$ agonist
Ondansetron	+++	0
Granisetron	+++	0
Tropisetron	++	0
Cisapride	0	++
Metoclopramide	+	++

0 no effect; +, ++, +++ definite effect.

Adverse effects

Metoclopramide crosses the blood-brain barrier and may cause extra-pyramidal reactions (see p.352); domperidone does not.

Cisapride is cardiotoxic at high plasma concentrations; it causes prolongation of the QT interval and predisposes to ventricular arrhythmias. The maximum recommended dose is 40 mg/24 h. Imidazole antifungal antibiotics prolong the halflife of cisapride and cause marked increases in plasma concentration (Box 14.A).

The warning in Box 14.A about a serious drug interaction between imidazole antifungals or certain antibiotics and cisapride is an example of responsible caution by the manufacturers. The original reports were of *ketoconazole* given in daily doses of 600–1200 mg in patients with prostate cancer. The interaction relates to inhibition of one of the liver cytochrome P450 enzymes. Partly because it is given in smaller doses, fluconazole has less effect on the enzyme than ketoconazole. The likelihood of this interaction occurring with fluconazole 50–100 mg o.d. is infinitesimal.

Box 14.A   Serious drug interaction with cisapride [modified from manufacturer's letter 11/95]

Rare cases of serious (occasionally fatal) cardiac arrhythmias, including ventricular arrhythmias and Torsade de Pointes associated with QT prolongation have been reported in patients taking cisapride in combination with *imidazole antifungals (flucon-azole, ketoconazole, itraconazole, miconazole), erythromycin or clarithromycin.* Some of these patients did not have known cardiac histories; most had been receiving multiple other medications and had pre-existing cardiac disease or risk factors for arrhythmias.

Concomitant administration of cisapride with oral or parenteral (but not topical) forms of imidazole antifungals, erythromycin or clarithromycin is now contra-indicated.

Psychotropics

Psychotropics are drugs whose primary use is to alter the patient's psychological state. They can be classified as

- neuroleptics/antipsychotics
- anxiolytic sedatives

- antidepressants

- psychostimulants

- psychodysleptics/hallucinogens.

Generally, smaller doses should be used in debilitated patients with advanced cancer than in physically fit patients, particularly if they are already receiving morphine or another psychotropic drug.

After an initial small test dose, the dose can be increased fairly quickly (e.g. every 2–3 days) until troublesome adverse effects appear or a satisfactory response is obtained.

There may be a need for a subsequent reduction in dose because of drug cumulation. As with analgesics, close supervision is essential particularly during the first few days.

A few patients respond paradoxically when prescribed psychotropics, e.g. diazepam (become more distressed) or amitriptyline (become wakeful and restless at night). Other patients derive little benefit from a benzodiazepine, e.g. diazepam, but are helped by a neuroleptic, e.g. haloperidol.

Psychostimulants have little place in palliative care despite their ability to enhance postoperative analgesia. For patients who complain of drowsiness, alternative measures should be considered (see p.74).

Cannabinoids are the only psychodysleptics which are used in palliative care. Like psychostimulants, they are of benefit only occasionally

- as an anti-emetic (at some centres in relation to chemotherapy)

- for dyspnoea (see p.152)

- for spasticity in multiple sclerosis.[9]

Neuroleptics

Neuroleptics are marketed primarily as antipsychotics and include the phenothiazines and the butyrophenones. In palliative care, however, they are used extensively as anti-emetics (see p.194). They act by blocking dopamine type 2 receptors in the brain and may cause extrapyramidal reactions (see p.352), and also hyperprolactinaemia. Phenothiazines also affect cholinergic, α-adrenergic, histaminergic, and serotonergic receptors.

Levomepromazine is the only phenothiazine with specific analgesic properties.[10] The use of chlorpromazine for malignant rectal tenesmoid pain has fallen into disrepute as alternative approaches to the management of neuropathic pain have been introduced and with the availability of spinal analgesia.

In chronic pain, the combination of a neuroleptic with an antidepressant is not more effective than treatment with an antidepressant alone.[11] The incidence of sedation is several times greater for the combination of morphine and chlorpromazine than for morphine alone.[12]

Neuroleptics are of benefit, however, in selected highly anxious patients overwhelmed by persisting pain and insomnia.[13] Benefit may also be seen in patients whose pain escalates with the onset of delirium (acute confusion) and who derive no benefit from increased doses of opioids.[14]

At Sobell House, haloperidol is the neuroleptic of choice (see p.331). The relative potencies of neuroleptics in psychotic patients serve as a guide for use in palliative care (Table 14.11).

Table 14.11   Pharmacokinetic data for selected neuroleptic drugs

Drugs	Halflife (h)	Oral bio-availability (%)	Equivalent oral dose (mg)[15]
Haloperidol[16]	12–36	60	3
Fluphenazine[17]	15	3	1–2
Trifluoperazine[18]	8–12	NK[a]	5
Prochlorperazine[19]	8[18][b]	15	?
Thioridazine[20]	6–40	–	100
Chlorpromazine[21,22]	7–15	10–25	100
Levomepromazine[23]	16–30	40	25–50

a   NK = not known

b   chronic administration.

Haloperidol

Properties and uses

- anti-emetic
- antipsychotic
- anxiolytic.

Limitations

- anticholinergic effects
- extrapyramidal reactions
- drowsiness.

General comments

- plasma halflife is 24 h +/– 12 h; generally given as a single dose nocte
- oral bio-availability = 60%
- extrapyramidal reactions more likely at daily doses of > 5 mg. Because these do not occur predictably, an antiparkinsonian drug should not be prescribed prophylactically
- anxiolytic of choice if a patient is hallucinating, paranoid, or in agitated delirium.

Haloperidol versus chlorpromazine

- less sedative
- less anticholinergic
- less cardiovascular effects
- more potent anti-emetic
- more extrapyramidal reactions.

Therapeutic guidelines

Haloperidol is available in solution, capsule (0.5 mg), tablet (1.5, 5, 10, 20 mg) and parenteral forms.

Anti-emetic

- for chemical/toxic causes of vomiting:
  1–1.5 mg stat and nocte (standard for morphine-induced vomiting)
  3–5 mg nocte if smaller dose not effective
  10–20 mg nocte, or in divided dosage, for chemotherapy-related vomiting and in some patients with renal failure
- as a potent dopamine type 2 antagonist, it is possible that haloperidol has a prokinetic effect comparable to domperidone, and might therefore correct gastric stasis induced by stress, anxiety or nausea from any cause (*see* p.325).

Antipsychotic

- 1.5–3 mg stat and nocte in the elderly
- 5 mg stat and nocte in younger patients or if poor response in the elderly
- 10–30 mg nocte (or in divided dosage) if poor response.

Anxiolytic

- 5 mg stat and nocte
- 10–20 mg nocte (or in divided dosage) if poor response.

Phenothiazines

Phenothiazines are classified according to chemical structure (Table 14.12). Thioridazine and levomepromazine are the only phenothiazines used at Sobell House.

Table 14.12 Classification of phenothiazines

Ethylamino derivatives Promethazine *Propylamino derivatives* Chlorpromazine Levomepromazine Promazine Alimemazine *Piperidine derivatives* Ethopropazine Thioridazine	*Piperazine derivatives* (halogenation of RI side chain) Fluphenazine Perphenazine Prochlorperazine Thiethylperazine Trifluoperazine

Properties and uses

- antipsychotic
- anti-emetic, particularly piperazine derivatives
- anxiolytic
- night sedative ⎫ particularly propylamino derivatives
- analgesic, *only levomepromazine* (*see* p.334)
- anti-sweating (*see* thioridazine, p.335).

Limitations

- anticholinergic effects
- drowsiness
- postural hypotension
- extrapyramidal reactions, particularly piperazines.

Therapeutic guidelines

Phenothiazines are manufactured in syrup, tablet, suppository and parenteral formulations but availability varies from country to country. Note

- plasma halflives of some phenothiazines show wide interpatient variation (*see* Table 14.11)

- most phenothiazines need to be given t.d.s. at most; sometimes just at bedtime

- generally, parenteral doses are several times smaller than oral doses (*see* Table 14.11)

- generally, parenteral administration should be IM because the SC route is too irritant

- prochlorperazine may be given by intermittent SC injection but, if it causes erythema or discomfort, give IM.

Levomepromazine

Properties and uses

- anti-emetic

- analgesic[10,24]

- antipsychotic

- neuroleptic sedative.

Levomepromazine is a broad-spectrum anti-emetic which is widely used as a second or third line agent in patients who fail to respond to more specific drugs (*see* p.197). Like chlorpromazine, it is a potent D_2- and α_1-receptor antagonist. In addition, it manifests potent $5HT_2$-receptor antagonism which probably accounts for both its anti-emetic potency and its analgesic effect.[25]

Limitations

- sedation, particularly with SC dose of $\geqslant 25$ mg/24 h

- dose-dependent postural hypotension

- limited range of preparations, i.e. tablet 25 mg, injection 25 mg/ml.

General comments

- plasma halflife 15–30 h; can generally be given as a single dose nocte

- oral bio-availability = 40%

- anti-emetic dose range typically 5–12.5 mg SC/24 h, sometimes 25–50 mg/ 24 h

- in the management of terminal agitation +/– delirium, doses may be much higher, ranging up to 200 mg/24 h and occasionally more[26]

- currently not often used as an analgesic but may be of benefit in a very distressed patient with severe pain unresponsive to other measures; doses comparable to those used for terminal agitation

- anecdotal evidence suggests that levomepromazine may relieve pruritus unresponsive to other measures (see p.251).[27]

Levomepromazine versus chlorpromazine

- more anti-emetic

- more sedative

- more postural hypotension

- analgesic.

Thioridazine

Uses

- antipsychotic

- night sedative

- anti-sweating.

Limitations

- limited range of preparations, i.e. tablets, suspensions and syrup

- no parenteral preparation available in the UK.

General comments

- plasma halflife is 6–40 h

- equipotent with chlorpromazine as an antipsychotic[15]

- used at Sobell House in preference to chlorpromazine when a neuroleptic more sedative than haloperidol is needed

- useful in patients with troublesome sweating not associated with infection, e.g. 25 mg nocte (see p.257).[28]

Thioridazine versus chlorpromazine

- less postural hypotension

- less extrapyramidal reactions

- less anti-emetic
- more anticholinergic.[29]

Benzodiazepines

Benzodiazepines are a group of anxiolytic sedative drugs with muscle relaxant and anticonvulsant properties (Table 14.13).

Although the relationship is nonlinear, the plasma halflives of a benzodiazepine and its pharmacologically active metabolites reflect the duration of action (Table 14.14; Figure 14.3). Those with long halflives

- can be used as anxiolytics o.d.
- tend to cumulate when given repeatedly
- are more likely to cause drowsiness and impaired psychomotor skills.

Table 14.13   Pharmacological properties of selected benzodiazepines[30]

Drug name	Anxiolytic	Night sedative	Muscle relaxant	Anticonvulsant
Diazepam	+++	+	+++	+++
Lorazepam	+++	+	+	+
Clonazepam	+	+++	+	+++
Nitrazepam	+	+++	+	+
Flunitrazepam	+	+++	+	+
Clorazepate	+	+	+	+
Chlordiazepoxide	+	+	0	+
Oxazepam	+++	+	0	0
Clobazam	+	0	0	+
Triazolam	0	+++	0	0
Temazepam	+	0[a]	0	0

Pharmacological activity: 0 minimal effect; + slight; ++ moderate; +++ marked.

a   the failure to demonstrate significant night sedative effect with temazepam emphasizes a limitation of the study, namely the restriction to one dose in volunteers.

Table 14.14 Classification of benzodiazepines

Short acting (halflife < 5 h)[a]	Intermediate acting (halflife 5–25 h)	Long acting (halflife > 25 h)
Midazolam	Flunitrazepam (22)	Chlordiazepoxide
Triazolam	Loprazolam (6–12)	Clonazepam
	Lorazepam (10–20)	Clorazepate
	Lormetazepam (11)	Diazepam
	Oxazepam (5–15)	Flurazepam
	Temazepam (8–15)	Nitrazepam

a halflife refers to the combined plasma halflives of the named drug and any pharmacologically active metabolites.

Clinical indications

- insomnia
- anxiety
- muscle tension/spasm
- myoclonus
- convulsions.

Routes of administration

- the oral route is best when used as a night sedative, anxiolytic or muscle relaxant
- diazepam is available as both a suppository and a rectal solution
- standard preparations of parenteral diazepam are oil-based and should not be given IM as absorption is slow and variable. IV diazepam may cause thrombophlebitis
- emulsified diazepam is preferable for IV administration but is more expensive

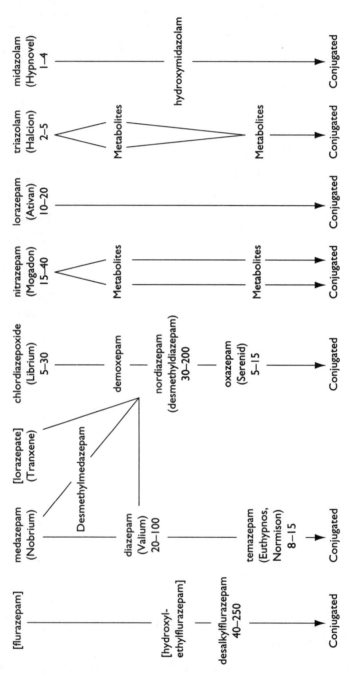

Figure 14.3 Metabolic pathways for selected benzodiazepines. Names in square brackets are drug precursors which do not reach the systemic circulation in clinically important amounts. Figures refer to plasma elimination halflives in hours. Lorazepam does not use the P450 hepatic metabolic pathway and avoids drug interactions relating to competitive inhibition of metabolism.

- IV lorazepam is less likely than diazepam to cause thrombophlebitis and respiratory depression but causes more amnesia. As it exhibits a variable delay between administration and onset of action, it is not recommended

- midazolam and flunitrazepam are water-soluble and can be given SC, IM and IV.

Therapeutic guidelines

It is important to be aware of the relative potency of the commonly used benzodiazepines (Table 14.15).

Table 14.15   Approximate equivalent anxiolytic sedative doses

Drug	Dose
Lorazepam	500 mcg
Diazepam	5 mg
Nitrazepam	5 mg
Temazepam	10 mg
Chlordiazepoxide	15 mg
Flurazepam	15 mg
Oxazepam	15 mg

Night sedative

- short acting drugs:
  midazolam is not available in tablet form in the UK (halflife = 1–4 h)
  triazolam is not available in the UK (halflife = 2–5 h)

- temazepam 10–40 mg, occasionally 60 mg, is widely used (halflife = 8–15 h)

- flunitrazepam is marketed as a night sedative 0.5–2 mg but its plasma halflife is 22 h.

For patients who feel oversedated in the morning, zopiclone or zolpidem should be used (*see* p.109).

Anxiolytic

- intermediate acting drugs:
  lorazepam 1–2 mg b.d.–t.d.s.
  temazepam 10 mg b.d.–t.d.s.

- long acting drugs:
  diazepam 2–20 mg nocte, occasionally more often (*see* p.309).

Muscle relaxant

- diazepam 2–20 mg nocte

- baclofen (*not* a benzodiazepine) is a useful alternative, particularly if anxiety is not an associated problem and if diazepam too sedative.

Anticonvulsant

- diazepam

- midazolam

- clonazepam.

Clonazepam is very potent and needs to be introduced in very small doses, e.g. 0.5 mg nocte, rising by 0.5 mg every 3–5 days up to 2–4 mg, and only occasionally more.

Diazepam

Properties and uses

- anxiolytic

- night sedative

- muscle relaxant

- anticonvulsant.

Diazepam is sometimes used as an adjuvant anti-emetic in patients receiving chemotherapy.

Limitations

- daytime drowsiness

- muscular flaccidity
- postural hypotension.

General comments

- plasma halflife 20–100 h; generally given once a day at *bedtime*. If patient does not sleep at night, daytime drowsiness more likely
- patients occasionally react paradoxically, i.e. become more distressed; if this happens, change to haloperidol or chlorpromazine
- diazepam acts faster PO or PR than IM because the standard preparation is oil-based; IV may cause thrombophlebitis
- if available, use diazepam oil-in-water emulsion (Diazemuls); this is less irritant.

Therapeutic guidelines

Initial dose depends on

- patient's previous experience of diazepam and other benzodiazepines
- intensity of distress
- urgency of relief.

The following doses are a guide

- 2 mg is useful and safe in the elderly
- 5 mg is the typical initial dose
- 10 mg is useful for severe distress, particularly in younger patients.

Repeat *hourly* until the desired effect is achieved, and then decide on an appropriate maintenance regimen.

Rectal diazepam is useful in a crisis or if the patient is moribund

- suppositories 10 mg
- rectal solution 5–10 mg in 2.5 ml
- parenteral formulation inserted through a cannula.

Lorazepam 1 mg tablets can be given SL as an alternative; this is equivalent to diazepam 10 mg.

Patterns of use

- as needed is the best initial way in the elderly, and for acute (possibly transient) episodes of severe anxiety
- regularly at bedtime is best for those with persistent anxiety – to be used as an adjunct to psychological measures; also if used for muscle spasm or general stiffness
- more than daily (e.g. 1000/1400, 2200 h or 1000, 1800, 2200 h) in agitated moribund patients to reduce the number of hours the patient is awake and distressed.

Midazolam

The main advantage of midazolam is that it is water-soluble and is miscible with most of the drugs commonly given by continuous SC infusion. It is also easier for IV injection.

Properties and uses

- anaesthetic induction agent
- sedative for minor procedures
- sedative for terminal agitation
- anticonvulsant.

Midazolam versus diazepam

In single doses

- for sedation, midazolam is 3 times as potent
- as an anticonvulsant, midazolam is twice as potent.

With multiple doses, diazepam will gain in potency because of its prolonged plasma halflife, i.e. 20–100 h versus 1–4 h for midazolam (but about 10 h when given by infusion).

Patterns of use

Typical doses for midazolam are shown in Table 14.16.

In terminal agitation, if the patient is not settled on 30 mg/24 h, introduce a neuroleptic before increasing the dose of midazolam further.

Table 14.16 Dose recommendations for SC midazolam

Indication	Stat dose	Initial infusion rate/24 h	Common range
Muscle relaxant Multifocal myoclonus	5 mg	10 mg	10–30 mg
Terminal agitation Anticonvulsant	10 mg	30 mg	30–60 mg

Antidepressants

There are many subtle differences between the actions of different anti-depressants. It is important to study the *Datasheet* and *National Formulary* when developing a prescribing policy for antidepressants in palliative care.

Tricyclics and SSRIs are the drugs of choice for the treatment of depression (Table 14.17). The tricyclic-related drugs, maprotiline and mianserin, are not used at Sobell House. Generally, MAOIs should be used only with specialist psychiatric advice. In severe depression which does not respond to drugs, electroconvulsive therapy (ECT) may be necessary.

Pharmacology

Tricyclic and related drugs have a range of actions (Table 14.18)

- blockade of re-uptake by presynaptic nerve terminals of:
    serotonin (5HT)
    norepinephrine

- receptor blockade:
    muscarinic cholinergic
    H_1-histaminergic
    α_1-adrenergic.

Table 14.17   Classification of antidepressants

Tricyclics Amitriptyline Clomipramine Desipramine Dothiepin Doxepin Imipramine Lofepramine Nortriptyline Trimipramine *Tricyclic-related* Maprotiline Mianserin *SSRIs* Fluoxetine Fluvoxamine Paroxetine Sertraline	*MAOIs* Phenelzine Isocarboxazid Tranylcypromine *RIMAs* Moclobemide *Other* Flupenthixol Tryptophan Lithium

The following should be noted

- sedation is related to blockade of the central H_1-histaminergic receptors

- hypotension is related to blockade of the α_1-adrenergic receptors

- H_1-histaminergic and α_1-adrenergic potency are closely correlated

- there is no correlation between anticholinergic potency and sedation, e.g. protriptyline is nonsedative but moderately anticholinergic

- sedative effects tend to be more common in physically ill patients, particularly if receiving other psycho-active drugs, including morphine

- the antidepressant effect of the tricyclics is related to the enhancement of the actions of norepinephrine and serotonin as neurotransmitters.

Selective serotonin re-uptake inhibitors (SSRIs)

As their name suggests, this group of antidepressants selectively blocks the presynaptic re-uptake of serotonin.[31] The elimination halflives of fluvoxamine, paroxetine and sertraline range from 15–30 h. The halflife of fluoxetine is about

Table 14.18 Pharmacological properties of some antidepressants[31]

Drug name	Type	Plasma halflife (h)	Norepinephrine uptake inhibition	Serotonin uptake inhibition	Anticholinergic effects	Sedative effects
Tricyclics						
Imipramine[a]	Tertiary amine	4–18	++	+++	++	++
Amitriptyline[b]	Tertiary amine	10–25	+	+++	+++	++
Clomipramine	Tertiary amine	16–20	+	+++	++	++
Nortriptyline	Secondary amine	13–93	+++	+	++	0
Desipramine	Secondary amine	12–61	+++	0	+	0
Protriptyline	Secondary amine	54–198	+++	++	++	0
Doxepin[c]	Tertiary amine	8–25	+	+	+++	++
Dothiepin	Tertiary amine	14–40	++	+	+	++

continued

Table 14.18 *continued*

Drug name	Type	Plasma halflife (h)	Norepinephrine uptake inhibition	Serotonin uptake inhibition	Anticholinergic effects	Sedative effects
Tricyclic-related						
Maprotiline[d]	Secondary amine	27–58	+++	+	+	+
Mianserin[e]	Tertiary amine	8–19	0	0	0	+
Trazodone[e]		4	0	+	0	+
Viloxazine	Secondary amine	2–5	+++	0	0	0

Pharmacological activity: 0 none; + slight; ++ moderate; +++ marked.

a metabolized to desipramine

b metabolized to nortriptyline

c metabolized to desmethylodoxepin (halflife 33–81 h)

d a bridged tricyclic

e inhibits presynaptic α_2-receptors.

2 days, and that of its active metabolite norfluoxetine is about 7 days. The longer action of fluoxetine is a disadvantage if adverse effects develop, if the patient takes an overdose, or if a drug which interacts with fluoxetine is substituted, e.g. a MAOI.

SSRIs are much less likely to cause sedation and anticholinergic effects than are the tricyclic antidepressants. They are also less likely to cause weight gain, confusion in the elderly, and cardiac arrhythmias and heart block in patients with heart disease. SSRIs, however, may cause extrapyramidal effects (*see* p.355).

Sertraline is the SSRI of choice at Sobell House. It is as effective as amitriptyline in treating depression with anxiety. The standard dose is 50 mg *in the morning* preferably after food; it is occasionally necessary to increase the dose to 100–200 mg. The antidepressant action of sertraline may be enhanced by sodium valproate.[32] Like other SSRIs it may cause an initial exacerbation of anxiety. It may also cause nausea and/or diarrhoea.

The manufacturer's data sheet states that sertraline should be avoided in patients with unstable epilepsy and that patients with controlled epilepsy should be carefully monitored. The drug should be discontinued in any patient who develops seizures.

Mianserin

Mianserin acts presynaptically by blocking α_2-adrenergic receptors. This results in increased norepinephrine release and turnover. Mianserin is about 2.5 times more potent than amitriptyline, i.e. mianserin 60 mg is equivalent to amitriptyline 150 mg. It is moderately sedative but is not anticholinergic.

Mianserin has occasionally been associated with agranulocytosis. This is generally reversible on stopping treatment. Most cases occur in the first month of treatment; the manufacturers recommend monthly blood counts for the first 3 months. Agranulocytosis is more common in the elderly and in patients with organic disease.

Mono-amine oxidase inhibitors (MAOIs)

There is little place for MAOIs in palliative care. A potentially fatal excitatory crisis may occur if tyramine-containing foods are eaten or certain drugs are prescribed concurrently, notably pethidine/meperidine (Table 14.19; Box 14.B). This interaction is precipitated by an increased concentration of cerebral serotonin. It occurs with pethidine, but not with other opioids.[33,34]

One report appears to implicate morphine.[35] It relates to a patient who regularly took a MAOI and trifluoperazine 20 mg daily, and who was given pre-operative promethazine 50 mg IM and morphine 1 mg IV followed by two

Table 14.19   Excitatory interaction with MAOIs

Tyramine-containing foods	Mono-amine-enhancing drugs
Cheese	Pethidine
Pickled herring	Other antidepressants
Broad bean pods	Reserpine

Meat or yeast extract
    Bovril
    Oxo
    Marmite
	Sympathomimetics (included in some proprietary cough mixtures)
	
	Levodopa

Alcohol
    red wine (white wine is safe)
    beer
	Tetrabenazine

Box 14.B   Excitatory interaction between pethidine and MAOIs

In patients taking a MAOI, the following may become apparent within minutes of the administration of a pethidine injection

- restlessness, excitability, possibly violent behaviour
- rigidity
- multifocal myoclonus +/– convulsions
- sweating and pyrexia
- cyanosis and stertorous respirations
- hypertension (and headache) or hypotension
- increased tendon reflexes, extensor plantar responses
- drowsiness, coma.

doses of morphine 2.5 mg IV. About 3 min after the third bolus, she became unresponsive and hypotensive (systolic pressure 160 → 40 mm Hg). The patient responded within 2 min to IV naloxone. This was *not* a MAOI excitatory crisis but, rather, a hypotensive response to IV morphine in someone chronically taking an α-adrenergic antagonist, i.e. trifluoperazine. Marked hypotension is always a risk following IV morphine, particularly in opioid-naive patients.

Therapeutic guidelines

Antidepressants are used to treat various symptoms in palliative care

- depression
- early morning insomnia
- nerve injury pain (*see* p.45)
- urgency of micturition (*see* p.224)
- urge incontinence
- nocturnal enuresis
- bladder spasms (*see* p.226).

The choice of antidepressant depends partly on the intended use. Table 14.18 provides a rational basis for prescribing. A few drugs cover all clinical needs, e.g.

- amitriptyline (sedative, marked anticholinergic effects)
- dothiepin (sedative, minimal anticholinergic effects)
- desipramine (nonsedative, minimal anticholinergic effects)
- paroxetine (nonsedative, no anticholinergic effects but may cause nausea).

Some centres use lofepramine; 70 mg is equivalent to amitriptyline 50 mg. It is less anticholinergic and less cardiotoxic in overdose.

Depressed cancer patients are often also anxious and the best results are generally obtained with a sedative drug, e.g. amitriptyline, dothiepin. A sedative antidepressant is also required to correct early morning insomnia.

Clomipramine is the tricyclic of choice for patients with depression associated with obsessional features.

For nerve injury pain and for bladder spasms and urgency caused by detrusor hyperreflexia, amitriptyline is a good choice.

All tricyclics can be given in a single dose at bedtime.

- if the patient experiences early morning drowsiness, or takes a long time settling at night, advise to take 1–2 h before bedtime
- anticholinergic cardiac effects are occasionally troublesome, but a cardiac history is not a contra-indication to careful use

- a small number of patients are stimulated by amitriptyline and experience insomnia, unpleasant vivid dreams, myoclonus and physical restlessness. In these patients, change to a SSRI or administer amitriptyline in the morning
- when an antidepressant is used to treat nerve injury pain, benefit may be seen as early as 3–5 days
- an antidepressant effect may also be seen as soon as this, although it commonly takes longer
- relatively small doses are often effective in relieving depression in debilitated cancer patients
- it is wise to commence with a small dose of a tricyclic in patients with advanced cancer, particularly if frail or elderly (Table 14.20).

Table 14.20   Dose escalation timetables for amitriptyline

Dose	Elderly frail/outpatient	Younger patient/inpatient
25 mg nocte	Week 1	Day 1
50 mg nocte	Week 2	Day 2–4
75 mg nocte	Week 3 + 4	Day 5–14
100 mg nocte	Week 5 + 6	Week 2
150 mg nocte	Week 7 + 8[a]	Week 3[a]

a   not often necessary in palliative care.

Hyoscine

Hyoscine (scopolamine) is an anticholinergic with smooth muscle relaxant (antispasmodic) and antisecretory properties. It is available as *hydrobromide* and *butylbromide* (Buscopan) salts. The latter is a quaternary salt and does not cross the blood-brain barrier. Unlike hyoscine *hydrobromide*, hyoscine *butylbromide* does not cause drowsiness, nor does it have a central anti-emetic action.

General comments

- hyoscine *butylbromide* is poorly absorbed PO. By this route it is of use only in intestinal colic

- repeated administration of hyoscine *hydrobromide* leads to cumulation and may result paradoxically in an agitated delirium. If this occurs, add diazepam or midazolam.

Preparations

Hyoscine butylbromide

- PO 10 mg

- SC 20 mg.

Hyoscine hydrobromide

- SL 0.3 mg (Quick Kwell)

- SC 0.4 mg, 0.6 mg

- transdermal patch 0.5 mg over 3 days.

If a SL preparation is required in the USA use *hyoscyamine* instead, e.g. 0.125 mg (Levsin). Hyoscyamine is the laevo-isomer of atropine. As the dextro-isomer is virtually inactive, hyoscyamine is approximately twice as potent as atropine.

Therapeutic guidelines

Injections of hyoscine *butylbromide* are cheaper than hyoscine *hydrobromide* and should generally be used in preference. The main indications are

- death rattle (*see* p.155)

- inoperable bowel obstruction (*see* p.201):
  to relieve colic
  as an antisecretory agent.

Hyoscine *hydrobromide* by any route and hyoscine *butylbromide* SC can also be used in other situations where an anticholinergic may be beneficial, e.g. sialorrhoea.

Despite a plasma halflife of about 8 h, the duration of antisecretory effect after a single dose in healthy volunteers is only about 1 h (butylbromide) and 2 h (hydrobromide). Thus, hyoscine is best given as a transdermal patch or by continuous SC infusion.

Anticholinergic effects

'Dry as a bone, blind as a bat, red as a beet, hot as a hare, mad as a hatter.'

Several drugs used in palliative care have anticholinergic (antimuscarinic) properties (Table 14.21).

Table 14.21   Anticholinergic drugs used in palliative care

Belladonna alkaloids
  atropine
  hyoscine
	Antihistamines
	  chlorphenamine
	  cyclizine
	  dimenhydrinate
	  promethazine

Glycopyrronium	

Neuroleptics
  butyrophenones
  (haloperidol, droperidol)
  phenothiazines
	Antispasmodics
	  mebeverine
	  oxybutynin
	  propantheline

Tricyclic antidepressants	

Anticholinergic effects may be a limiting factor in symptom management. The concurrent use of two anticholinergics should be avoided, if possible. A list of anticholinergic effects is given in Table 14.22.

Drug-induced movement disorders

Drug-induced movement disorders encompass

- extrapyramidal reactions:
    parkinsonism
    acute dystonia
    acute akathisia
    tardive dyskinesia

- malignant neuroleptic syndrome.

Table 14.22   Anticholinergic effects

Visual

Mydriasis
Loss of accommodation $\Big\}$ blurred vision

Cardiovascular

Palpitations
Extrasystoles $\Big\}$ also related to norepinephrine potentiation and a
Arrhythmias quinidine-like action

Gastro-intestinal

Dry mouth
Heartburn (reduced tone in lower oesophageal sphincter)
Constipation

Urinary tract

Hesitancy of micturition
Retention of urine

The features of the various syndromes are listed in Table 14.23. Extrapyramidal reactions are caused mostly by drugs which block dopamine receptors in the CNS; this includes all neuroleptics and metoclopramide.[36] Other drugs have also been implicated (Table 14.24), including antidepressants and ondansetron.[37,38,39]

High potency neuroleptics possess a greater affinity for dopamine receptors and a lower affinity for cholinergic receptors than low potency neuroleptics. They therefore cause a greater inbalance between dopamine and acetylcholine, and are more likely to cause extrapyramidal reactions. Thus haloperidol is high risk but, for example, levomepromazine is low risk. More extrapyramidal reactions occur at higher doses of any potentially causal drug. There is probably also a genetic factor.

To explain the mechanism by which antidepressants and ondansetron cause extrapyramidal reactions, a 'four neurone model' has been proposed which includes 5HT- and GABA-receptors.[40]

Parkinsonism

Parkinsonism develops in up to 40% of patients treated long term with neuroleptics. It develops at any stage after commencement of treatment, although

Table 14.23 Movement disorders associated with dopamine-receptor antagonists[41]

Parkinsonism	Acute dystonias	Acute akathisia	Tardive dyskinesia	Neuroleptic malignant syndrome
Coarse resting tremor of limbs, head, mouth and/or tongue	*One or more of*	*One or more of*	Exposure to neuroleptic medication for ≥ 3 months (1 month if 60+ years of age)	Severe muscle rigidity and Pyrexia + *Two or more of*
Muscular rigidity (cogwheel or leadpipe)	Abnormal positioning of head and neck (retrocollis, torticollis)	Fidgety movements or swinging of legs	Involuntary movement of tongue, jaw, trunk or limbs	Tremor Sweating Mutism
Bradykinesia (notably of face)	Spasms of jaw muscles (trismus, gaping, grimacing)	Rocking from foot to foot when standing	choreiform (rapid, jerky, nonrepetitive)	Dysphagia Incontinence Drowsiness
Sialorrhoea (drooling)	Tongue dysfunction (dysarthria, protrusion)	Pacing to relieve restlessness	athetoid (slow, sinuous, continual)	Tachycardia Elevated/labile blood pressure
Shuffling gait	Dysphagia	Inability to sit or stand still for several minutes	rhythmic (stereotypic)	Leucocytosis Evidence of muscle injury (myoglobinuria, raised plasma creatine kinase concentration)
	Laryngo-pharyngeal spasm			
	Dysphonia			
	Eyes deviated up, down, or sideways ('oculogyric crisis')			
	Abnormal positioning of limbs or trunk			

Table 14.24   Drugs which may cause extrapyramidal effects[38,42]

Palliative care	General

Neuroleptics
  haloperidol
  phenothiazines
	Diltiazem

	Fenfluramine
Metoclopramide	5-Hydroxytryptophan
Ondansetron	Lithium

Antidepressants[a]
  tricyclics
  SSRIs
	Methyldopa

	Methysergide
Carbamazepine	Reserpine

a   all classes of antidepressants have been implicated except RIMAs.

not generally before the second week. It is most common in the over 60s. Although generally symmetrical, there may be asymmetry in the early stages.

Regular rhythmic tremors of the hands, head, mouth or tongue with a frequency of 8–12 cps may be induced by a wide range of drugs (Table 14.25). These must not be confused with drug-induced parkinsonism. A drug-induced postural tremor is generally absent at rest but intensifies when the affected part is used or held in a sustained position, e.g. hands outstretched, mouth held open. In contrast, the tremor of drug-induced parkinsonism is typically

Table 14.25   Drug-induced (nonparkinsonian) postural tremor[43]

Anticonvulsants
  sodium valproate
	Methylxanthines
	  caffeine
	  aminophylline
	  theophylline

Antidepressants
  SSRIs
  tricyclics	

	Neuroleptics
	  butyrophenones
	  phenothiazines

β-Adrenoceptors
  salbutamol
  salmeterol	

	Psychostimulants
	  dexamphetamine
	  methylphenidate

Lithium	

lower in frequency, worse at rest, suppressed during intentional movements, and is typically associated with rigidity and bradykinesia (Table 14.23).

Treatment

Use an anticholinergic antiparkinsonian drug

- benzatropine 1–2 mg IV/IM → 2 mg PO o.d.–b.d. *or*
- procyclidine 5–10 mg IV/IM → 2.5–5 mg PO t.d.s.
- orphenadrine 50–100 mg PO b.d. is a useful alternative.

Acute dystonia

Acute dystonias occur in up to 10% of patients treated with neuroleptics. They develop abruptly within days of starting treatment, and are accompanied by anxiety (Table 14.23). They are most common in young adults.

Treatment

- benzatropine 1–2 mg or procyclidine 5–10 mg IV/IM for immediate relief. Benefit is seen within 10 min; peak effect within 30 min. If necessary, repeat after 30 min
- continue treatment with a standard oral anticholinergic antiparkinsonian drug (*see above*)
- some centres use IV/IM diphenhydramine 20–50 mg, followed by 25–50 mg b.d.–q.d.s.
- consider discontinuing or reducing dose of causal drug
- if caused by metoclopramide, substitute domperidone.

Acute akathisia

Akathisia is a form of motor restlessness in which the subject is compelled to pace up and down or to change the body position frequently (Table 14.23). It is most common in the 16–50 age range. It occurs in up to 20% of patients receiving neuroleptics. It can develop within days of starting treatment. If the drug is continued, it may progress to parkinsonism. Haloperidol and prochlorperazine carry the highest risk.[44] It is uncommon for metoclopramide to cause akathisia. Concurrent administration of morphine or sodium valproate may be additional risk factors.[44]

Treatment

- consider reducing dose of causal drug
- switch to a neuroleptic with more anticholinergic activity
- prescribe an anticholinergic antiparkinsonian drug (as for acute dystonia)
- if only partial response, add diazepam 5 mg nocte
- alternatively, prescribe a *lipophilic* β-adrenoceptor antagonist; i.e. propranolol 10–40 mg b.d. or metoprolol 50–100 mg b.d.
- in resistant cases, discontinue causal drug.

Akathisia responds less well to antiparkinsonian drugs than drug-induced parkinsonism and dystonias. Propranolol, a highly lipophilic nonselective β-adrenoceptor antagonist, and metoprolol, a lipophilic β_1-adrenoceptor antagonist, are equally effective. In contrast, atenolol, a *hydrophilic* β_1-adrenoceptor antagonist, has no effect.

Tardive dyskinesia

Tardive (late) dyskinesia is caused by the long term administration of drugs that block dopamine receptors, particularly D_2-receptors. It occurs in 20% of patients receiving a neuroleptic for more than 3 months. Women, the elderly and those on high doses, e.g. chlorpromazine 300 mg/day, are most commonly affected.

Tardive dyskinesia typically manifests as involuntary stereotyped chewing movements of the tongue and orofacial muscles. The involuntary movements are made worse by anxiety and reduced by drowsiness and during sleep. Tardive dyskinesia seldom causes subjective distress, unless associated with akathisia. This is seen in 25% of cases.

In younger patients, tardive dyskinesia may present as abnormal positioning of the limbs and tonic contractions of the neck and trunk muscles causing torticollis, lordosis or scoliosis. In younger patients, tardive dyskinesia may occur if neuroleptic treatment is stopped abruptly but not if tailed off gradually.

Early diagnosis

'Open your mouth and stick out your tongue.'

The following indicate a developing tardive dyskinesia

- worm-like movements of the tongue
- inability to protrude tongue for more than a few seconds.

Treatment

- withdrawal of the causal agent leads to resolution in 30% in 3 months and a further 40% in 5 years; sometimes irreversible particularly in the elderly

- often responds poorly to drug therapy; anticholinergic antiparkinsonian drugs may exacerbate

- tetrabenazine – depletes presynaptic biogenic amine stores and blocks postsynaptic dopamine receptors. Best not used in depressed patients. Start with 12.5 mg t.d.s. → 25 mg t.d.s.; increase dose slowly to avoid troublesome hypotension

- reserpine – depletes presynaptic biogenic amine stores. May be used in place of tetrabenazine; causes similar adverse effects

- levodopa – may produce long term benefit after causing initial deterioration

- GABA antagonists – baclofen, sodium valproate, diazepam and clonazepam have all been tried with inconsistent results

- increase the dose of the causal drug – paradoxically, this may help but should be considered only in desperation.

Neuroleptic malignant syndrome

Neuroleptic malignant syndrome occurs in 1–2% of patients receiving a neuroleptic, particularly in young adults; two thirds of cases occur < 1 week after starting treatment.[45] It is more likely to occur in patients also receiving lithium.

The essential features of neuroleptic malignant syndrome are fever and muscle rigidity associated with some of the following: tremor, sweating, mutism, dysphagia, incontinence, drowsiness, tachycardia, elevated or labile blood pressure. Leucocytosis and evidence of muscle injury, i.e. myoglobinuria and raised plasma creatine kinase concentration, are laboratory features.

Treatment generally comprises

- discontinuation of the causal drug

- prescription of a muscle relaxant.

In severe cases, bromocriptine (a dopamine agonist) has been used. Death occurs in up to 20% of cases, most commonly as a result of respiratory failure.

References

1 Swartz SL and Dluhy RG (1978) Corticosteroids: clinical pharmacology and therapeutic use. *Current Therapeutics.* **Sept**: 145–170.

2 Rotstein J and Good RA (1957) Steroid pseudorheumatism. *AMA Archives of Internal Medicine.* **99**: 545–555.

3 Chalk JB *et al.* (1984) Phenytoin impairs the bio-availability of dexamethasone in neurological and neurosurgical patients. *Journal of Neurology, Neurosurgery and Psychiatry.* **47**: 1087.

4 Pokorny C *et al.* (1985) Comparison of an antacid/dimethicone mixture and an alginate/antacid mixture in the treatment of oesophagitis. *Gut.* **26**: A574.

5 Debinski HS and Kamm MA (1994) New treatments for neuromuscular disorders of the gastrointestinal tract. *Gastrointestinal Journal Club.* **2**: 2–11.

6 Schuurkes JAJ *et al.* (1986) Stimulation of gastroduodenal motor activity: dopaminergic and cholinergic modulation. *Drug Development Research.* **8**: 233–241.

7 McHugh S *et al.* (1992) Cisapride versus metoclopramide: an acute study in diabetic gastroparesis. *Digestive Diseases and Science.* **37**: 997–1001.

8 Fumagalli I and Hammer B (1994) Cisapride versus metoclopramide in the treatment of functional dyspepsia: a double-blind comparative trial. *Scandinavian Journal of Gastroenterology.* **29**: 33–37.

9 Martyn CN *et al.* (1995) Nabilone in the treatment of multiple sclerosis. *Lancet.* **345**: 579.

10 Bonica JJ and Halpern LM (1972) Analgesics. In: Modell W (ed) *Drugs of Choice 1972–1973.* CV Mosby, St Louis. pp 185–217.

11 Getto CJ *et al.* (1987) Antidepressants and chronic nonmalignant pain: a review. *Journal of Pain and Symptom Management.* **2**: 9–18.

12 Houde RW (1966) On assaying analgesics in man. In: Knighton RS, Dumke PR (eds) *Pain.* Little Brown, Boston. pp 183–196.

13 Maltebie A and Cavenar J (1977) Haloperidol and analgesia: case reports. *Military Medicine.* **142**: 946–948.

14 Coyle N *et al.* (1994) Delirium as a contributing factor to 'crescendo' pain: three case reports. *Journal of Pain and Symptom Management.* **9**: 44–47.

15 Foster P (1989) Neuroleptic equivalence. *Pharmaceutical Journal.* **Sept 30**: 431–432.

16 Data Sheet: haloperidol (1996) ABPI *Compendium of Data Sheet and Summaries of Product Characteristics 1996–1997.* Datapharm Publications, London. pp 449–450.

17 Koytchev R *et al.* (1996) Absolute bioavailability of oral immediate and slow release fluphenazine in healthy volunteers. *European Journal of Clinical Pharmacology.* **51**: 183–187.

18 Smith Kline Beecham Pharmaceuticals (1997) Personal Communication.

19 Dahl SG and Strandjord RE (1977) Pharmacokinetics of chlorpromazine after single and chronic dosage. *Clinical Pharmacology and Therapeutics.* **21**: 437–445.

20 Reynolds JEF (1996) Thioridazine. In: Martindale. *The Extra Pharmacopoeia.* (31st edn) Royal Pharmaceutical Society, London. pp 738–739.

21 Yeung PKF *et al.* (1993) Pharmacokinetics of chlorpromazine and key metabolites. *European Journal of Clinical Pharmacology.* **45**: 563–569.

22 Koytchev R *et al.* (1994) Absolute bioavailability of chlorpromazine, promazine and promethazine. *Arzneimittel-Forschung.* **44**: 121–125.

23 Dahl SG (1975) Pharmacokinetics of methotrimeprazine after single and multiple doses. *Clinical Pharmacology and Therapeutics.* **19**: 435–442.

24 Beaver W *et al.* (1966) A comparison of the analgesic effects of methotrimeprazine and morphine in patients with cancer. *Clinical Pharmacology and Therapeutics.* **5**: 436–446.

25 Twycross R *et al.* (1997) The use of low dose levomepromazine (methotrimeprazine) in the management of nausea and vomiting. *Progress in Palliative Care.* **5** (2): 49–53.

26 Johnson I and Patterson S (1992) Drugs used in combination in the syringe driver: a survey of hospice practice. *Palliative Medicine.* **6**: 125–130.

27 Closs SP (1997) Pruritus and methotrimeprazine. Personal communication.

28 Regnard C (1996) Use of low dose thioridazine to control sweating in advanced cancer. *Palliative Medicine.* **10**: 78–79.

29 Axelsson R and Martensson E (1976) Serum concentration and elimination from serum of thioridazine in psychiatric patients. *Current Therapeutic Research.* **19**: 242–265.

30 Ansseau M *et al.* (1984) Methodology required to show clinical differences between benzodiazepines. *Current Medical Research and Opinion.* **8** (Suppl 4): 108–113.

31 Ashton CH (1989) *Brain Systems, Disorders and Psychotropic Drugs.* Oxford Medical Publications, Oxford.

32 Dave M (1995) Antidepressant augmentation with valproate. *Depression.* **3**: 157–158.

33 Browne B and Linter S (1987) Monoamine oxidase inhibitors and narcotic analgesics. A critical review of the implications for treatment. *British Journal of Psychiatry.* **151**: 210–212.

34 Stockley IH (1994) Monoamine oxidase inhibitors and morphine or methadone. In: Stockley IH (ed) *Drug Interactions.* (3rd edn) Blackwell Scientific Publications, Oxford. pp 642–644.

35 Barry BJ (1979) Adverse effects of MAO inhibitors with narcotics reversed with naloxone. *Anaesthesia and Intensive Care.* **7**: 194.

36 Tonda ME and Guthrie SK (1994) Treatment of acute neuroleptic-induced movement disorders. *Pharmacotherapy.* **14** (5): 543–560.

37 Zubenko GS *et al.* (1987) Antidepressant-related akathisia. *Journal of Clinical Psychopharmacology.* **7**: 254–257.

38 Arya DK (1994) Extra-pyramidal symptoms with selective serotonin reuptake inhibitors. *British Journal of Psychiatry.* **165**: 728–733.

39 Mathews HG and Tancil CG (1996) Extrapyramidal reaction caused by ondansetron. *Annals of Pharmacotherapy.* **30**: 196.

40 Hamilton MS and Opler LA (1992) Akathisia, suicidality, and fluoxetine. *Journal of Clinical Psychiatry.* **53**: 401–406.

41 American Psychiatric Association (1994) Neuroleptic-induced movement disorders. In: *Diagnostic and Statistical Manual of Mental Disorders.* (4th edn) (DSM-IV). American Psychiatric Association, New York. pp 736–751.

42 Anonymous (1994) Drug-induced extrapyramidal reactions. *Current Problems in Pharmacovigilance.* **20**: 15–16.

43 American Psychiatric Association (1994) Medication-induced postural tremor. In: *Diagnostic and Statistical Manual of Mental Disorders.* (4th edn) (DSM-IV). American Psychiatric Association, New York. pp 749–751.

44 Gattera JA *et al.* (1994) A retrospective study of risk factors of akathisia in terminally ill patients. *Journal of Pain and Symptom Management.* **9**: 454–461.

45 Launer M (1996) Selected side-effects: 17. Dopamine-receptor antagonists and movement disorders. *Prescribers' Journal.* **36**: 37–41.

Index